# DMSO FOR ADULTS AND SENIORS

### THE BIBLE FOR NATURAL HEALING

### MINIMIZE CHRONIC PAIN AND INFLAMMATION INCREASE ENERGY AND VITALITY WITH PROTOCOLS

### MT VESSEL

# CONTENTS

| | |
|---|---|
| *Introduction* | 7 |
| 1. UNDERSTANDING DMSO: THE FOUNDATION OF NATURAL HEALING | 11 |
| The Science Behind DMSO: Simplified for Everyone | 11 |
| DMSO and Its Role in Reducing Inflammation | 13 |
| Exploring DMSO's Anti-Aging Properties | 15 |
| The History and Evolution of DMSO in Medicine | 17 |
| Debunking Myths: What DMSO Can and Cannot Do | 19 |
| 2. SAFE AND EFFECTIVE DMSO APPLICATION TECHNIQUES | 23 |
| Topical Use of DMSO: A Step-by-Step Guide | 23 |
| DMSO Dosage: Finding the Right Balance | 25 |
| Oral Intake of DMSO: What You Need to Know | 27 |
| Inhalation Methods: Breathing New Life with DMSO | 29 |
| Avoiding Common Mistakes in the DMSO Application | 31 |
| 3. ADDRESSING PAIN AND MOBILITY CHALLENGES | 33 |
| Chronic Pain Management: A Natural Approach with DMSO | 36 |
| Overcoming Limited Mobility with DMSO | 38 |
| Success Stories: Real-Life Experiences in Pain Relief | 39 |
| Comparing DMSO to Conventional Pain Treatments | 41 |
| 4. ENHANCING SKIN HEALTH AND OVERCOMING SENSITIVITIES | 45 |
| Addressing Skin Sensitivity: Precautions and Tips | 47 |
| DMSO for Wound Healing and Recovery | 49 |
| Navigating Allergies and Skin Reactions | 51 |

5. INTEGRATIVE APPROACHES: COMBINING
   DMSO WITH OTHER NATURAL REMEDIES                57
   Complementary Therapies: Enhancing DMSO's
   Benefits                                         60
   Anti-Inflammatory Diets: Boosting DMSO's
   Effectiveness                                    62
   Yoga and Exercise: Promoting Mobility and Healing
   with DMSO                                        65

6. OVERCOMING SKEPTICISM: THE EVIDENCE
   FOR DMSO                                         69
   Scientific Studies: What the Research Says
   About DMSO                                       71
   Addressing Concerns: Safety and Efficacy of DMSO 74
   Busting the "Too Good to Be True" Myth           76

7. FINANCIAL ACCESSIBILITY AND QUALITY
   ASSURANCE                                        79
   Cost-Effective Solutions: Making DMSO Affordable 79
   Choosing High-Quality DMSO Products              82
   Comparing Costs: DMSO vs. Traditional Treatments 84
   DIY Health Practices: Economical Use of DMSO     86

8. COMMUNITY AND SUPPORT: BUILDING
   CONNECTIONS                                      89
   Sharing Experiences: Testimonials and Tips       92
   Community Workshops: Learning and Growing
   Together                                         93
   Building a Support System: Family and Friends
   Involvement                                      95

9. ENHANCING OVERALL WELLNESS WITH DMSO           99
   Mind-Body Connection: Stress Management
   with DMSO                                        101
   Long-Term Health Goals: Using DMSO for
   Longevity                                        103
   Holistic Health: Embracing a Balanced Lifestyle  105

10. THE FUTURE OF DMSO AND EMERGING
    THERAPIES                                       109
    DMSO and Emerging Therapies: What's Next?       111
    Exploring Nicotine: A Hidden Bombshell for Focus
    and Energy                                      113

| | |
|---|---|
| DMSO in the Next Decade: Predictions and Possibilities | 115 |
| Preparing for the Future: Staying Informed and Engaged | 117 |
| *Conclusion* | 121 |
| *References* | 127 |

# INTRODUCTION

Hello, I'm your author. I know that's a little weird for an introduction, but I believe a little bio will set the stage and allow you to see my motivation for this book. I was in the Air Force for 8 active years and 8 years active reserves. While I was a reservist, I was also a general contractor in Atlanta, Ga. The construction business itself takes a toll on your body, as you may expect, and it was no different for me. While I was active in the Air Force, at 24(1985), a back injury set the stage for years of pain and discomfort. During the time between 1989 and 1994, I moved to Florida and became a framing and trim carpentry contractor. It was during that time that I damaged all but one lower lumbar vertebra. In 1995, I progressed into the supervisor role for a major production builder in the area and gave my back a rest, but never got away from the pain my injuries had caused.

In 1996, having been a chain smoker for about 11 out of the preceding 15 years, I was diagnosed with bladder cancer and sent home to get my "affairs in order." During the next 3 1/2 years, they harvested (my term) no less than 20 tumors from my bladder through a catheter. In 1999, I changed urologists and got a doctor who cared about me for who I was. He said to me after the first tumor ectomy, "Mark, are you still smoking? It's ok if you are. I have 2 kids to get through college, and your procedures will pay for all their tuition". In my head, I said, "hell no, I'm not; I have my kids to support." Then, I proceeded to explain how hard it was to quit in my current line of work. He explained Wellbutrin to me and prescribed it. In 8 days, by a miracle, I was an instant non-smoker and have been a non-smoker for the last 25 years—no more tumors after that moment. In a management role at the time, I just lived with the pain and drank quite a bit to numb it, but I slept terribly and always woke up feeling terrible and still in pain.

In 2014, while on a mission trip to Guatemala, life took an unexpected turn. There, leading a group of younger adults to build a house for a family in need, I suffered a severe injury to the last vertebra in my lower lumbar. The pain was intense and debilitating, a reminder of my earlier struggles with chronic pain and health challenges. After getting back home over a week later, the best surgeon in the area told me I'd have a 50/50 chance of playing golf again after surgery, or I could stay off of it for a year, and it would just about heal itself. He further stated that he didn't think I'd stay off it, but it was my choice. I stayed off of it, and it healed. I played golf again but continued to live with chronic pain and inflammation. These experiences shaped my journey and fueled my quest for healing. They are also examples of life, and there are millions of us around the world. My story exemplifies there are good and harmful medicines, but we have to be in tune with our bodies and what is happening around us, no matter where we are geographically.

The mission trip injury was a catalyst. It led me to physical massage, legal CBD, nicotine, and DMSO, a compound that would change my life. My introduction to DMSO was fortuitous. A trusted friend shared their knowledge, piquing my curiosity. I dived into research, spending countless hours studying its properties and potential. I was thorough, cautious, and open-minded. Through experimentation and the support of close friends, I found a path to being pain-free, something I hadn't experienced in over 35 years.

This book is the culmination of that journey. It is my way of sharing the knowledge and insights gained along the way. My goal is simple: to educate you about DMSO, its benefits, and how to use it safely. This compound is a powerful tool for minimizing pain and inflammation. When used correctly, it can boost energy and vitality. I aim to provide practical guidance, helping you integrate DMSO with other natural remedies for a holistic approach to your good health. I'll provide you with a list of links and references. Furthermore, I encourage you to research yourself. Few people today care more about you than they do about their profit. I'm sorry, but call it what it is, A Problem.

I envision this book as a resource for all adults. It is designed to empower you with knowledge to make informed decisions about your health and wellness. I want to demystify DMSO so that it is understandable to those who may read it now and in the future. With the right tools, you can take control of your health journey. With good resources and Information, you can help friends and family.

As you explore these pages, you'll find intriguing topics beyond DMSO. For instance, the power of using DMSO with other natural substances. These discussions aim to broaden your perspective and spark curiosity. They encourage you to think about health in new and innovative ways. That said, I encourage you to be open-minded on this journey and study the research while you fight off the urge to fall back on false information that the public has been conditioned to believe. Alternative remedies are real. They have been around for decades and centuries with positive results. Tested and proven beyond numerous medicines and vaccines on the market today, with practically no side effects. Isn't it suspicious to you that any substance that can't be patented by those in control for the purpose of making enormous sums of money is classified as bad and dangerous by those same entities? Watch for yourself. I'm not a conspiracist, but the facts are plain if you know what and where to look for them.

Throughout this book, I desire to connect with you. I understand the challenges of living with chronic pain and the quest for relief, which drives my passion for sharing practical solutions. My experiences are not unique; many face similar health struggles. I offer this book as a beacon of hope and a source of practical advice. I must warn you that you will see some redundancy about safety and handling, please don't be discouraged. This book is set up so that people may use it repeatedly with quick reference to what they need without reading it all over again, so I have listed some things once more each time they are warranted. Your safety, in all of this great information, is my utmost concern.

In closing, this introduction sets the stage for a transformative health journey. Grounded in personal experience, practical knowledge, and extensive research, this book invites readers to explore the potential of DMSO as a natural remedy. Let us embark on this journey together, discovering new paths to health and wellness.

# 1

# UNDERSTANDING DMSO: THE FOUNDATION OF NATURAL HEALING

Understanding DMSO is like discovering a well-kept secret in a world where the search for natural healing is more prominent than ever. This chapter aims to clarify the science behind DMSO, a compound that has become a cornerstone of alternative health practices. You might wonder how a simple liquid can impact health so profoundly. It was this very curiosity that led me to explore DMSO, and it's this knowledge that I now share with you. By breaking down the complexities of DMSO, you'll gain insight into why it stands out among natural remedies.

## THE SCIENCE BEHIND DMSO: SIMPLIFIED FOR EVERYONE

DMSO, or dimethyl sulfoxide, might sound complex, but its essence is straightforward. This colorless liquid is an organosulfur compound, which means it's derived from sulfur, a fundamental element found in nature. DMSO uniquely dissolves polar and nonpolar compounds, making it **highly versatile as a polar aprotic solvent**. This characteristic is why DMSO can mix with many organic solvents and even **water**. DMSO's "high polarity" sets it apart, which allows it to interact efficiently with **biological membranes**, enhancing its ability to penetrate the skin and reach underlying tissues. This ability makes it an effective medium for transporting small molecules directly through the skin to other body parts.

Once DMSO enters the body, its interaction is remarkable. The compound facilitates the transport of small molecules across cell membranes, acting much like a courier delivering a package. This ability to enhance cellular permeability is crucial, allowing compounds that might otherwise remain on the surface to penetrate deeper. This feature boosts the effectiveness of medications or supplements applied with DMSO and enables the body to absorb them more efficiently. As a result, DMSO is often used in transdermal drug delivery, an area where its unique properties shine. It has been stated that DMSO does not accumulate in the body; it is depleted, and its remnants are disposed of through normal biological systems.

DMSO's biocompatibility with human tissue makes it particularly special among natural remedies. This means it can be used safely on or in the body without causing harm when used correctly. Its low toxicity is another significant advantage. While many chemical compounds can be harsh or damaging, DMSO is gentle, making it suitable for various applications. This characteristic has led to its use in multiple medical treatments, underscoring its value as a natural remedy. For example, it prolongs the viability of organs being transported to transplant recipients.

The scientific consensus on DMSO is evolving, but current research clearly shows that it holds substantial promise. The FDA has approved DMSO for specific medical applications, such as treating interstitial cystitis, a chronic bladder condition. This approval reflects the compound's safety and effectiveness in managing specific health issues. Moreover, ongoing studies continue to explore its potential in pain and inflammation management. Researchers are investigating how DMSO can be applied to alleviate conditions like arthritis, where traditional treatments might not suffice.

Understanding DMSO's capabilities involves recognizing its potential and limitations. The dialogue surrounding DMSO grows as science progresses, offering new insights and applications. This chapter serves as a gateway to understanding how DMSO can be a part of your wellness routine. Whether you're exploring it for its pain-relieving properties or its broader health benefits, DMSO stands as a testament to the power of nature in healing. As we delve into its science, you will see how this humble compound might hold the key to unlocking new levels of health and vitality.

## DMSO AND ITS ROLE IN REDUCING INFLAMMATION

Inflammation is a natural response by the body, often a sign that it's working to heal itself. Yet, when inflammation persists or becomes chronic, it can lead to pain and further health complications, for example, **Diabetes**. DMSO steps into this scenario as a potential ally, renowned for its anti-inflammatory properties. At a cellular level, DMSO works by inhibiting pro-inflammatory cytokines, which are proteins that signal inflammation in the body. These cytokines, when overactive, contribute to swelling, pain, and redness. By dampening these signals, DMSO helps reduce inflammation, offering relief. Moreover, DMSO plays a role in reducing oxidative stress. This stress occurs when there's an imbalance between free radicals and antioxidants in the body, leading to cell damage. By mitigating oxidative stress, DMSO alleviates inflammation and supports overall cellular health. I have witnessed this personally.

Several studies and clinical trials back the effectiveness of DMSO in managing inflammation. For instance, research involving arthritis patients has shown promising results. Patients reported reduced swelling and pain, with some experiencing improved mobility after consistent DMSO application. These clinical findings provide a solid foundation for DMSO's credibility as a treatment option. Another study examined DMSO's impact on reducing inflammation in sports-related injuries, revealing that athletes experienced quicker recovery times and less pain when DMSO was applied. Such evidence underscores the potential of **DMSO as a versatile anti-inflammatory** agent. The data from these trials not only highlights DMSO's therapeutic effects but also positions it as a viable alternative to conventional treatments.

When compared to traditional anti-inflammatory medications, such as non-steroidal anti-inflammatory drugs Novocaine or Procaine (NSAIDs), DMSO offers distinct advantages. While NSAIDs are commonly prescribed for pain and inflammation, they can lead to gastrointestinal issues and other side effects when used long-term. In contrast, DMSO presents fewer gastrointestinal side effects, making it a more beneficial option for most. However, it's essential to acknowledge that DMSO is not without its own set of issues, though they are miniscule. Some users report a garlic-like taste or odor after application, a minor inconvenience compared to the more severe side effects of NSAIDs. Despite this, the benefits of DMSO outweigh these minor concerns, especially for those seeking a more natural approach to inflammation management. Remember, **inflammation** is almost always felt as **pain.**

Beyond its traditional applications, DMSO is being explored for innovative uses. In the realm of sports injuries, DMSO is gaining traction for its ability to reduce inflammation and expedite recovery. Athletes and trainers increasingly consider DMSO as part of their injury management protocols. Furthermore, its potential to reduce post-surgical inflammation is being investigated. Patients recovering from surgery may benefit from DMSO's anti-inflammatory properties, which reduce swelling and accelerate healing times. These emerging uses highlight the versatility of DMSO as a therapeutic agent, expanding its relevance in both conventional and alternative medicine spheres.

DMSO presents a compelling option for those navigating the complexities of inflammation and seeking relief. Its unique properties, supported by clinical research, offer a pathway to managing inflammation with fewer side effects than many conventional treatments. Whether dealing with arthritis, recovering from an injury, or exploring ways to support post-surgical healing, DMSO's potential applications are diverse and promising. As research continues to unfold, the role of DMSO in inflammation management is likely to expand, offering hope and relief to those who need it most.

EXPLORING DMSO'S ANTI-AGING PROPERTIES

Aging is an inevitable part of life, yet the quest for youthful vitality persists across generations. DMSO emerges as a compelling candidate in the realm of skin health and anti-aging. This compound may contribute to healthier skin by stimulating collagen synthesis. Collagen, a protein responsible for skin elasticity and firmness, naturally diminishes over time, leading to wrinkles and sagging. By promoting collagen production, DMSO can help maintain the skin's structural integrity, potentially reducing the visible signs of aging. Additionally, DMSO's moisturizing effects cannot be understated. It allows the skin to retain moisture, which is crucial for maintaining a plump, smooth complexion. This hydration helps soften fine lines and wrinkles, giving the skin a more youthful appearance. At the same time, helping it to be more healthy at the cellular level.

In the realm of beauty and skincare, DMSO's applications are diverse. It is often used topically for wrinkle reduction. By applying DMSO directly to the skin, individuals can target specific areas prone to aging, such as the face and neck. Its ability to penetrate profoundly ensures that the beneficial effects reach the underlying layers where they are most needed. Additionally, DMSO can be combined with other skin-enhancing substances, such as vitamin C or hyaluronic acid, to amplify its effects. This combination approach allows for a more comprehensive skincare regimen, simultaneously addressing multiple aspects of skin health.

The scientific support for these claims is growing. Studies have observed notable improvements in skin elasticity, a key indicator of youthful skin, with DMSO use. These findings suggest that DMSO can effectively support skin health by enhancing elasticity and reducing the appearance of wrinkles. In cosmetic dermatology, clinical observations have further reinforced the potential of DMSO. Dermatologists have reported positive outcomes in patients using DMSO, citing skin texture and tone improvements. While more research is needed to understand the breadth of DMSO's anti-aging properties fully, the current evidence is promising.

Beyond skin-deep benefits, DMSO plays a significant role in cellular rejuvenation. Think of it as a facilitator of the body's internal repair systems. At the cellular level, DMSO promotes repair mechanisms that combat the wear and tear associated with aging. This includes enhancing the body's natural ability to regenerate cells and tissues, potentially slowing aging. Furthermore, DMSO boasts antioxidant properties that counteract free radicals. These unstable molecules contribute to aging and cellular damage. By neutralizing free radicals, DMSO helps protect cells from oxidative stress, a major factor in the aging process. This cellular support extends beyond the skin, benefiting overall health and vitality.

DMSO offers an intriguing option for those exploring ways to maintain a youthful appearance. Its ability to stimulate collagen synthesis, moisturize the skin, and protect against cellular damage positions it as a versatile tool in the fight against aging. DMSO is a natural compound that aligns with the growing preference for holistic and non-invasive beauty solutions. Whether used alone or in combination with other skincare ingredients, DMSO presents an opportunity to enhance skin health in a natural and effective way. As scientific exploration continues, the role of DMSO in anti-aging is likely to expand, offering new insights into its potential benefits.

## THE HISTORY AND EVOLUTION OF DMSO IN MEDICINE

The story of DMSO begins in the 19th century when the world was on the brink of an industrial revolution and scientific discovery. In this era, Russian scientist Alexander Zaytsev first synthesized dimethyl sulfoxide in 1866, laying the groundwork for what would become a significant compound in both industrial and medical fields. Initially, DMSO found its place as a solvent in various industrial applications due to its ability to dissolve a wide range of substances. This versatility made it a staple in laboratories and industries, used for everything from chemical reactions to the manufacturing of microelectronic devices.

However, the transition from industrial use to medical acceptance was not straightforward. The potential of DMSO as a medical compound was recognized much later when researchers began exploring its effects on biological systems—the shift from merely a solvent to a compound with therapeutic promise involved rigorous research and numerous challenges. One of the major hurdles was regulatory approval, as the medical community scrutinized its safety and efficacy. The FDA's approval process presented a significant barrier, requiring extensive clinical trials and evidence. Yet, despite these challenges, DMSO slowly gained recognition for its potential benefits, particularly in pain and inflammation management, where traditional treatments often fell short.

The 1960s marked a pivotal moment in DMSO's medical history, with major clinical trials exploring its efficacy in various conditions. These studies laid the foundation for the breakthroughs that would follow. One of the key developments was its application in pain management, where DMSO demonstrated significant potential. Patients experienced relief from chronic pain conditions, leading to increased interest and further research. These clinical trials were not without controversy, as some results were met with skepticism. However, they paved the way for broader acceptance and understanding of DMSO's therapeutic capabilities.

Today, DMSO stands at the intersection of traditional and complementary medicine, with its current status reflecting a blend of historical legacy and modern innovation. Researchers continue investigating its potential in new medical applications, exploring neuroprotection and regenerative medicine. The growing acceptance of DMSO in complementary medicine highlights a shift towards integrating natural compounds with conventional treatments. This evolution reflects a broader trend in healthcare, where patients and practitioners seek holistic health approaches. As research progresses, the prospects for DMSO expand, offering new possibilities for its use in diverse medical fields.

The journey of DMSO from an industrial solvent to a respected medical compound is a testament to the power of scientific exploration and persistence. Its history is rich with discoveries and challenges, each contributing to its current status. As we look to the future, the potential of DMSO remains vast, with researchers and practitioners poised to uncover new applications and benefits. The narrative of DMSO is not just about a chemical compound; it is about the ongoing quest for understanding and improving human health. Through continued research and innovation, DMSO's role in medicine is set to grow, offering hope and solutions to those seeking natural and effective health interventions.

## DEBUNKING MYTHS: WHAT DMSO CAN AND CANNOT DO

DMSO has not escaped the clutches of myths and misconceptions as with many natural remedies. One of the most persistent is the belief that DMSO is a miracle cure for many ailments. While DMSO has significant potential, it is not a panacea. Some claim it can cure everything from cancer to chronic pain without the need for traditional medical treatments. This exaggerated view is not only misleading but also potentially dangerous. Understanding what DMSO can realistically achieve is crucial. It's essential to recognize that while DMSO can alleviate specific symptoms and improve quality of life, it should not replace conventional medical treatments prescribed by healthcare professionals. It is an adjunct, not a substitute.

Another common myth concerns DMSO's safety profile. Some believe that because it is a natural compound, it is inherently safe in all circumstances. While DMSO is generally safe when used correctly, misuse can lead to complications. It is crucial to use DMSO cautiously, following appropriate guidelines and dosages. Like any treatment, natural or man-made, DMSO is not free from risks. Potential harm can occur, mainly if DMSO is applied to large areas of skin or used in high concentrations and/or volumes. These risks underscore the importance of informed use and consultation with a Holistic or Naturopathic Physician. They can provide guidance tailored to your specific health needs, ensuring that DMSO is used effectively and safely. Most family physicians are not keen on substances not made by big pharma, which has been my experience. So beware and be careful.

Understanding DMSO's limitations is equally essential. There are conditions in which DMSO might offer little to no benefit. For instance, while DMSO can help manage certain types of pain and inflammation, it is ineffective against all forms of disease or discomfort. It cannot cure systemic illnesses or replace the need for medical interventions that address underlying health issues. Recognizing these limitations allows for realistic expectations and more effective use of DMSO within a broader health strategy.

Using it based on scientific evidence is essential to fully appreciate DMSO's potential. While anecdotal success stories can be inspiring, they should be balanced with scientific research and clinical data. The importance of evidence-based practice cannot be overstated. Consulting with Naturopathic Physicians ensures that DMSO is incorporated into your health regimen to complement other treatments and therapies. This approach maximizes benefits and minimizes potential risks, leading to a more holistic and effective health strategy.

As we dispel myths and clarify truths, it becomes clear that DMSO offers substantial benefits when used wisely. It is a tool that requires understanding and respect. By recognizing its capabilities and limitations, you can make informed choices that support your health goals. This knowledge empowers you to use DMSO effectively, ensuring it contributes positively to your wellness journey. As you continue to explore the pages ahead, keep an open mind and a discerning eye, ready to embrace the possibilities that DMSO presents.

2

# SAFE AND EFFECTIVE DMSO APPLICATION TECHNIQUES

Imagine a tool in your wellness kit that has the potential to alleviate pain and inflammation with just a simple application to the skin. For many, DMSO has become that tool. Its topical use is one of the most straightforward and accessible methods for experiencing its benefits. However, like any tool, it requires proper handling to unlock its full potential. The journey to discovering these benefits begins with understanding the nuances of its application. My relief from years of chronic pain started with mastering these simple yet essential techniques, and now I share them with you to guide you on your path to improved health. So far, I've found all the products I needed on Amazon.com.

TOPICAL USE OF DMSO: A STEP-BY-STEP GUIDE

Applying DMSO topically starts with cleanliness. Before you begin, ensure that the skin is thoroughly cleansed. This step is crucial because clean skin facilitates better absorption and minimizes the risk of irritation. Use mild soap and water, and ensure the area is dry before proceeding. Once the skin is prepared, it's time to consider the dilution. The concentration of DMSO should be appropriate for the condition you're treating. For general use, a 70% DMSO solution mixed with 30% distilled water is commonly recommended, but a lower concentration might be preferable for more sensitive applications.

A patch test is a prudent step before you commit to widespread use. Apply a small amount of the diluted solution to a discreet skin area, like the inner arm, and wait 24 hours to observe any reaction. This test helps ensure that your skin tolerates DMSO well. Remember, every individual's skin reacts differently, and what works for one person might not work for another. If irritation occurs, adjusting the dilution or consulting a healthcare professional for guidance may be necessary.

Application is not just about applying the solution; it's about how you apply it. Use clean hands or sterile cotton pads to spread the solution over the area. This ensures that you aren't introducing any contaminants that could affect the skin. Gently massage the solution into the skin, allowing it to absorb naturally. For certain conditions, covering the area with a breathable bandage can help enhance absorption and keep the area clean. This method is beneficial if you're applying DMSO to a joint or muscle area you use frequently throughout the day.

Choosing the right conditions for application is equally important. DMSO works best when applied to small, localized areas with the most needed effects. Avoid applying it to sensitive or damaged skin unless a healthcare professional advises otherwise. The reason for this caution is that DMSO's ability to penetrate deeply can sometimes cause irritation or discomfort if the skin isn't intact. Monitoring the application area for any signs of irritation, such as redness or itching, is essential. If you notice any adverse reactions, discontinue use and seek medical advice.

# SAFE AND EFFECTIVE DMSO APPLICATION TECHNIQUES | 25

*Practical Checklist for Topical Application*

- **Clean the skin**: Use mild soap and water.
- **Choose the right dilution**: Start with a 70% DMSO solution unless otherwise advised.
- **Apply with care**: Use clean hands or sterile pads.
- **Consider covering**: Use a breathable bandage if needed.
- **Conduct a patch test**: Test on a small area before broader use.
- **Monitor reactions**: Watch for redness or irritation.

This checklist serves as a practical guide to using DMSO effectively and safely. By following these steps, you can maximize the benefits of DMSO while minimizing potential risks. Remember, the goal is not only to apply DMSO but to do so with the care and attention that ensures the best outcomes for your health and well-being.

## DMSO DOSAGE: FINDING THE RIGHT BALANCE

When it comes to using DMSO effectively, **understanding the importance of dosage cannot be overstated.** It's the difference between achieving the desired therapeutic effects and encountering unwanted side effects. Dosage varies significantly based on the treated condition, making it crucial to tailor your approach. For skin conditions, lower concentrations are generally sufficient. These can address issues like minor inflammation or localized discomfort without overwhelming the skin. Conversely, higher concentrations might be necessary for addressing joint pain or more severe inflammatory conditions requiring deeper tissue penetration. This flexibility in dosing allows you to customize DMSO use to your specific needs, optimizing its effectiveness.

Determining the right dosage involves several factors, each playing a role in how DMSO interacts with your body. The severity of symptoms is a primary consideration. Mild symptoms may only need a gentle touch of DMSO, while more intense pain or inflammation could require a stronger concentration. Individual tolerance also plays a significant part. Some people respond well to lower doses, experiencing relief with minimal application, while others may need a higher dose to achieve the same effect. This variability underscores the importance of starting with a conservative dose and gradually adjusting it as you observe how your body reacts. It's a process of careful observation and adaptation, ensuring you find the best balance for you.

However, it's important to emphasize the risks associated with improper dosage. Overusing DMSO can lead to skin damage, manifesting as irritation or burns if applied too liberally or frequently. This risk highlights the need for careful management, ensuring that you respect the potency of DMSO. Systemic absorption is another concern at high doses. When too much DMSO enters the bloodstream, it can lead to unintended effects, including potential interactions with other medications. This is particularly significant for those with existing medical conditions or those taking other treatments, as it could complicate their health regimen. Therefore, maintaining a thoughtful and cautious approach to dosage is not just advisable; it's necessary. If needed, contact a Natural or Holistic physician for professional guidance.

While navigating the complexities of DMSO dosage, keeping a few guiding principles in mind is beneficial. Begin with the lowest effective concentration, allowing your body to adjust and respond. Monitor your symptoms and any changes in your condition, noting improvements or adverse effects. Adjust the dosage incrementally, giving your body time to adapt to each change. This methodical approach helps prevent overuse and maximizes the therapeutic benefits of DMSO. It's a practice grounded in patience and attentiveness, ensuring that you achieve the best possible outcomes for your health and well-being. We highly recommend journaling all your notes.

## ORAL INTAKE OF DMSO: WHAT YOU NEED TO KNOW

Exploring the internal use of DMSO opens another dimension of its potential. When considering oral intake, weighing the potential benefits against the possible drawbacks is essential. One of the primary advantages of consuming DMSO orally is its ability to address systemic inflammation. This method allows DMSO to work from within, reaching areas that topical application might miss. For some, this has meant significant relief from conditions marked by widespread inflammation, such as chronic arthritis or certain autoimmune disorders. However, the internal route is not without its challenges. The most notable risk is gastrointestinal irritation. DMSO, when ingested, can sometimes cause discomfort in the digestive tract. Symptoms might include an upset stomach or mild nausea, particularly if taken in higher doses or without proper dilution. Understanding the risk is crucial for making informed decisions about whether oral DMSO is right for you.

Safe practices are imperative when ingesting DMSO. The starting point is dilution. Always mix DMSO with water or juice to reduce the concentration and minimize potential irritation. This makes it gentler on the stomach and helps with palatability, as DMSO has a distinctive taste that not everyone finds pleasant. It's wise to begin with a low dose (I started with 25% DMSO and 75% MCT from coconut oil), allowing your body time to adjust to this new supplement. Gradually increase the dosage as your tolerance grows, paying close attention to how your body responds. This incremental approach reduces the likelihood of adverse effects and helps identify the optimal dose for your needs. Another critical aspect of oral DMSO use is timing. Some find it beneficial to take it on an empty stomach, while others prefer it with food to further mitigate any gastric discomfort. Observing how your body reacts in different situations will guide you in finding the best method for your circumstances.

One cannot overstate the importance of consulting a healthcare provider before starting oral DMSO. This is particularly vital if you are taking other medications, as DMSO can interact with them. Such interactions might alter the effectiveness of your medications or exacerbate side effects. Your healthcare provider can offer tailored advice based on your medical history and current prescriptions, ensuring that you use DMSO safely. This step is not just about safety; it's about optimizing the benefits of DMSO for your unique health profile. A professional's insight can make all the difference in how you incorporate this treatment into your broader health regimen. Additionally, regular check-ins with your healthcare provider can help monitor your progress and make any necessary adjustments to your dosage or method of intake.

The potential of oral DMSO is illustrated through real-life examples. Consider a case where an individual with chronic inflammation found significant improvement in their symptoms through oral DMSO. After consulting a healthcare provider, this person began with a carefully measured dose and gradually increased it over time. The result was not only a reduction in inflammation but also an improvement in overall vitality and energy levels. While this is just one example, it underscores the potential of DMSO when used thoughtfully and with guidance. Such stories offer hope and inspiration, showing that oral DMSO can be a valuable tool in managing systemic health issues with the right approach. These accounts serve as reminders that while

DMSO is powerful, its success lies in its respectful and informed use.

## INHALATION METHODS: BREATHING NEW LIFE WITH DMSO

While DMSO is widely recognized for its topical applications, its potential extends into the realm of inhalation, offering a different avenue for its therapeutic use. Inhalation might initially seem unconventional, yet it presents intriguing possibilities, particularly for respiratory conditions. Imagine the ability to directly target respiratory issues, providing relief where needed most. The premise of using DMSO in this way lies in its ability to enhance the delivery of therapeutic agents through the respiratory tract. This method allows DMSO to reach areas that might be inaccessible through other forms of administration, potentially offering swift relief from respiratory discomfort and inflammation.

The process of inhaling DMSO requires careful attention to detail to ensure safety and effectiveness. To begin, a nebulizer is typically used to facilitate controlled compound delivery. This device converts liquid DMSO into a fine mist, allowing it to be inhaled deeply into the lungs. To prepare the solution for inhalation, DMSO is diluted with saline. This dilution is crucial, as it reduces the concentration to a safe level for the delicate tissues of the respiratory tract. Once diluted, the solution is placed in the nebulizer, ready for inhalation. This method allows for precise control over the dosage and ensures that the DMSO is evenly distributed throughout the respiratory system.

Safety is paramount when using DMSO via inhalation. Proper ventilation is necessary to prevent the accumulation of vapors, which can cause irritation if inhaled in high concentrations. Ensure the area is well-ventilated during the process, reducing the risk of inadvertently inhaling a higher dose than intended. Additionally, be mindful of who is present during the inhalation process. Some individuals, especially those with sensitivities or allergies, might react adversely. It's best to conduct this practice in isolation or with aware and consenting individuals. Monitoring for any signs of discomfort or adverse reactions is critical, and if any occur, cease the process immediately and seek medical advice.

The benefits of DMSO inhalation are compelling, yet they come with limitations. It is not a universal solution and may not be suitable for everyone. Anyone, especially those who are pregnant or breastfeeding, should consult a healthcare provider before considering this method. However, inhalation may offer rapid relief from respiratory issues, such as bronchitis or asthma, for those without contraindications. The direct delivery to the lungs allows DMSO to act swiftly, reducing inflammation and easing breathing. It is important, however, to approach this method with realistic expectations. While it can provide quick relief, it is not a cure-all and should be used as part of a comprehensive treatment plan tailored to individual needs by experienced Physicians.

Inhalation offers a unique opportunity to explore DMSO's capabilities beyond traditional applications. It highlights this compound's versatility and potential to address respiratory concerns effectively. Understanding and respecting this method's nuances opens the door to new possibilities in managing health challenges. As with any treatment, informed use and professional guidance are the cornerstones of safety and success.

# SAFE AND EFFECTIVE DMSO APPLICATION TECHNIQUES | 31

## AVOIDING COMMON MISTAKES IN THE DMSO APPLICATION

Navigating the world of DMSO applications can be straightforward, but it requires a keen awareness to avoid common pitfalls. A frequent error many people encounter is the temptation to use undiluted DMSO directly on sensitive skin. This approach can lead to irritation or worse, as DMSO is a potent substance that should be treated respectfully. Always remember that DMSO's strength is best harnessed when appropriately diluted. Ignoring dilution guidelines can lead to discomfort and undermine the compound's potential benefits. Similarly, bypassing a patch test before full application is another critical mistake. This simple step, often overlooked, can prevent unnecessary reactions by ensuring your skin tolerates the solution well. It's a small precaution that pays significant dividends in providing a safe experience with DMSO.

To prevent these missteps, starting with lower concentrations is advisable. By easing into DMSO use, you give your body the chance to acclimate, reducing the likelihood of adverse reactions. Consulting with professionals, whether they are healthcare providers or experienced users, can also provide invaluable guidance. Their insight can help you navigate the initial stages of DMSO use, ensuring you apply it correctly and understand its effects. This guidance can become a cornerstone of your DMSO routine, providing the confidence to use this compound effectively and safely.

When mistakes occur, they can significantly impact treatment outcomes. Misusing DMSO can delay healing, as irritation or adverse reactions may sideline your progress. These setbacks can be frustrating, especially when they are avoidable with some care and preparation. Moreover, improper use increases the risk of side effects, ranging from mild discomfort to more severe skin reactions. Understanding these potential outcomes emphasizes the importance of adhering to recommended practices. It's a reminder that while DMSO is powerful, its benefits are best realized through careful, informed use. Learning from these experiences, whether firsthand or through others, is crucial in refining your approach.

To illustrate, consider the stories of those who have navigated these challenges. One individual, eager to experience the benefits of DMSO, applied it undiluted and without testing. The result was a harsh skin reaction that took weeks to resolve. From this, they learned the importance of dilution and patience, adjusting their approach with much better results. Another user, skeptical of the need for a patch test, experienced unexpected irritation. This experience taught them the value of precaution, leading to more informed and safer use of DMSO thereafter. These real-life accounts serve as powerful reminders of the lessons that come from trial and error. They highlight the importance of preparation and adaptability in achieving health goals with DMSO.

As we close this chapter, remember that avoiding common mistakes in DMSO applications is more than following steps. It's about understanding the compound, respecting its capabilities, and adapting to its nuances. By integrating these practices, you will ensure effective and safe use and unlock the full potential of DMSO in your health regimen. The next chapter will delve into the practical side of managing pain and mobility challenges, exploring how DMSO can enhance your quality of life.

# 3

# ADDRESSING PAIN AND MOBILITY CHALLENGES

Imagine waking up in the morning, eager to embrace the day, only to be greeted by the familiar ache of arthritis. This pain is not just a physical sensation; it's an unwelcome companion that influences every movement and decision. Some people will remember those mornings vividly, the stiffness in their joints reminding them of their limitations. Yet, amid this challenge lies a promising ally—DMSO, a tool that can transform how we manage arthritis. Understanding its potential begins with how it addresses the core issues of joint pain and inflammation, offering a pathway to reclaiming your mobility and independence.

Arthritis, a condition characterized by inflammation and joint pain, is a common adversary in many lives. DMSO steps in with a unique ability to reduce joint inflammation through cellular mechanisms. When applied, DMSO penetrates deeply into the skin, reaching the affected joints and working at a cellular level. It suppresses the production of pro-inflammatory cytokines, chemicals that signal inflammation in the body. By reducing these signals, DMSO alleviates the swelling and pain associated with arthritis. Its action improves synovial fluid circulation, the lubricant that cushions and protects your joints. Enhanced circulation means less friction and more freedom of movement, allowing you to engage in activities you once enjoyed without the constant reminder of pain.

Applying DMSO for arthritis requires a thoughtful approach to maximize its benefits. Begin by preparing a proper dilution, especially for sensitive joint areas. A common starting point is a 70% DMSO solution mixed with 30% distilled water, though some may find a weaker dilution more suitable. Using a clean applicator, gently apply the solution to the affected joints, ensuring even coverage. The frequency of application is crucial for chronic conditions. Consistent use, often twice daily, can enhance its effects, gradually reducing inflammation and improving mobility. Patience is key; give your body time to respond to this new regimen. The transformation may not be immediate, but with persistence, you will likely notice a positive shift in how your joints feel and function.

Regular use of DMSO can lead to long-term benefits, offering a horizon of hope for those with arthritis. Over time, you may experience increased joint flexibility and a greater range of motion. These improvements can fundamentally change your daily life, allowing you to move easily and confidently. Additionally, as your symptoms diminish, there is potential to reduce dependency on medication. This shift lessens the burden of side effects and empowers you to take control of your health. The goal is to support your body's natural healing processes, paving the way for sustained joint health and vitality.

Integrating DMSO into your arthritis management plan is about more than just application; it's about embracing a holistic approach to wellness. Complementary strategies can enhance

DMSO's effectiveness. Consider combining its use with physical therapy exercises tailored to your needs. These exercises can strengthen the muscles around your joints, providing additional support and stability. Dietary changes are another valuable component. Embracing an anti-inflammatory diet rich in omega-3 fatty acids and antioxidants can bolster your body's defenses against inflammation, working in tandem with DMSO to promote overall joint health.

*Practical Tips for Arthritis Management*

- **Dilution**: Start with a 70% DMSO solution for sensitive joints.
- **Application**: Apply twice daily with a clean applicator for best results.
- **Physical Therapy**: Incorporate exercises to support joint strength.
- **Dietary Adjustments**: Focus on anti-inflammatory foods to aid healing.

These practical tips serve as a roadmap to navigating arthritis with greater ease. By integrating these elements into your routine, you create a comprehensive strategy that supports your joints and your entire well-being. As you explore these options, remember that the journey to improved mobility is personal and unique. Embrace the possibilities and move forward confidently with the knowledge and tools to regain control over your arthritis.

## CHRONIC PAIN MANAGEMENT: A NATURAL APPROACH WITH DMSO

Living with chronic pain can feel like navigating an endless maze of discomfort and limitations. Yet, among the many potential solutions, DMSO stands out for its unique ability to modulate pain signals. When applied, DMSO penetrates deeply to reach nerve endings, influencing the transmission of pain signals. Through a process known as modulation, it alters the way nerves communicate pain to your brain, reducing the intensity of the sensation. This means that the relentless ache of chronic pain conditions like fibromyalgia and chronic back pain can be softened, allowing you a respite from their grasp. The way DMSO works is akin to adjusting the volume on a radio—while the signal is still present, it's much less intrusive.

Fibromyalgia sufferers often endure widespread pain and tenderness. DMSO offers a glimmer of hope, potentially easing the severity of these symptoms. By modulating pain pathways, it addresses the nerve hyperactivity that characterizes this condition. Similarly, for those dealing with chronic back pain, DMSO can provide targeted relief. Its ability to penetrate profoundly means it can reach areas of inflammation and nerve irritation, offering soothing relief. These conditions, known for their persistent nature, may find a worthy opponent in DMSO, which provides a natural alternative to conventional pain relief methods. Its role in reducing nerve pain is particularly beneficial, as it addresses the root of the discomfort rather than simply masking the symptoms.

For those embarking on a regimen of DMSO for chronic pain, consistency is key. Start with a daily application, focusing on the areas where pain is most pronounced. Apply a diluted solution, typically a 70% concentration, ensuring the skin is clean and dry. This practice allows DMSO to work effectively, directly benefiting the affected nerves and tissues. Monitor your progress closely. Note any pain level or frequency changes, adjusting the dosage as needed. Some may find relief with a single daily application, while others might benefit from more frequent use. Be patient; chronic pain did not develop overnight, and finding the right balance with DMSO may take time.

Managing chronic pain with DMSO also involves overcoming certain challenges. Initial discomfort or skin reactions are not uncommon, especially as your body adjusts to the compound. If this occurs, consider reducing the concentration or frequency of application. These adjustments can help your skin acclimate without compromising the treatment's effectiveness. Another hurdle is managing expectations. It's important to approach DMSO with realistic goals, understanding that while it can provide relief, it may not eliminate pain entirely. Patience is crucial. Allow your body time to respond, and remember that improvement often comes gradually. These challenges are part of the process, and with careful navigation, the potential for significant pain reduction is within reach.

As you integrate DMSO into your daily routine, consider it a companion in your journey toward managing chronic pain. Its natural properties offer a gentle yet effective means of addressing the complexities of nerve-related discomfort. Embrace the process, and give yourself grace as you explore this path to relief. Chronic pain management is multifaceted, and DMSO adds a valuable tool to your arsenal. Its ability to modulate pain signals presents a promising avenue for those seeking a natural and less invasive approach to pain relief.

## OVERCOMING LIMITED MOBILITY WITH DMSO

Navigating the challenges of limited mobility can often feel daunting, impacting both the body and mind. However, DMSO offers a promising avenue to enhance physical movement by targeting muscle stiffness and improving circulation in affected areas. When applied, DMSO acts as a gentle relaxant, easing muscle tension that often leads to restricted movement. This relaxation alleviates discomfort and encourages better blood flow. Enhanced circulation is crucial as it brings essential nutrients and oxygen to tissues, promoting healing and reducing the sensation of tightness. With regular use, DMSO can gradually loosen those stubborn knots that inhibit your freedom of movement, offering a path to more fluid and comfortable mobility.

To maximize the benefits of DMSO, pairing its application with specific exercises can amplify its effects. Gentle yoga routines, for instance, are a wonderful complement. They promote flexibility and balance, allowing your joints to move more freely and comfortably. Yoga poses such as the cat-cow stretch or seated forward bend can be particularly effective when combined with DMSO, as they gently encourage the body to release tension while the compound softens rigidity. Additionally, incorporating range-of-motion exercises can further support your mobility goals. Movements like shoulder circles or ankle rotations can keep your joints lubricated and agile. These exercises create a harmonious balance between physical activity and DMSO's therapeutic properties when performed consistently. Remember, "motion is lotion."

The benefits of improved mobility extend beyond the physical realm, significantly impacting mental health. As movement becomes easier, so does the return of confidence and independence. Daily tasks without assistance or discomfort can uplift your spirits, fostering a sense of accomplishment and autonomy. This newfound freedom can also reduce anxiety related to mobility limitations. The fear of falling or injuring oneself often diminishes as you regain control over your body, allowing you to engage more fully in life. This psychological uplift is an integral part of the healing process, reinforcing the physical improvements achieved with DMSO and exercise.

To maintain these gains, consistency is key. Regular application of DMSO, combined with daily or weekly exercise routines, can sustain and even enhance the progress you've made. Set a schedule that works for you, encouraging steady improvement without overwhelming your body. Equally important is maintaining open communication with your healthcare provider. Regular check-ins can ensure that your plan remains effective and safe, allowing for adjustments as needed. Your provider can offer valuable insights and monitor changes, ensuring your mobility journey continues positively. These strategies, when combined, create a robust framework for overcoming limited mobility, empowering you to live with greater ease and joy.

## SUCCESS STORIES: REAL-LIFE EXPERIENCES IN PAIN RELIEF

Imagine a life where every step feels like a battle, each movement a test of endurance. For many, this is the reality of living with arthritis, a condition that turns routine activities into monumental tasks. Take, for example, the story of Helen, a senior who spent years grappling with the limitations imposed by arthritis. Once nimble and skilled, her hands became stiff and painful, affecting her ability to enjoy her favorite pastimes like knitting and gardening. After being introduced to DMSO, Helen found a gradual return of her mobility. She began applying it consistently, following the recommended guidelines for dilution and frequency.

Over time, her joints felt less inflamed, the pain subsiding enough to allow her to resume her hobbies. The transformation was not instantaneous, but her patience paid off, illustrating DMSO's profound impact on regaining one's quality of life.

Another compelling narrative comes from Mark, a middle-aged man whose life was overshadowed by chronic back pain. The pain was a constant companion, affecting his work and personal life. Searching for alternatives, he discovered DMSO and incorporated it into his daily routine. By diligently applying it to his lower back, Mark noticed a significant decrease in pain intensity. This allowed him to engage in activities he had long avoided, such as playing with his children and participating in sports. His experience highlights the broad applicability of DMSO, offering relief not just to the elderly but also to those in their prime. Through Mark's journey, the potential of DMSO as a natural pain relief option becomes evident, showing how it can unlock new opportunities for those willing to explore its benefits.

Across these stories, a common thread emerges: consistency and adherence to application guidelines play crucial roles in successful DMSO use. Helen and Mark both found success by committing to regular application, allowing their bodies to adjust and respond. This consistency ensures that DMSO can work effectively, minimizing inflammation and pain over time. Their stories also emphasize the importance of combining DMSO with other wellness practices. Helen paired her DMSO regimen with gentle stretching exercises, while Mark incorporated mindfulness techniques to manage stress. This holistic approach enhances the overall effectiveness of DMSO, creating a synergy that amplifies healing.

Feedback from these experiences provides valuable lessons for others considering DMSO. Patience is paramount. Both Helen and Mark learned that progress takes time and that immediate results are rare. Instead, gradual improvement marked their paths, underscoring the necessity of perseverance. Finding the right balance of DMSO concentration was also key. Each individual's needs and tolerances vary, and adjusting the dilution to suit one's specific condition can make a significant difference. Their stories remind us that while DMSO is powerful, its success lies in its careful and informed use. These accounts serve as beacons of hope and guidance, offering practical insights for those seeking to alleviate pain and enhance mobility through natural means.

## COMPARING DMSO TO CONVENTIONAL PAIN TREATMENTS

Pain management is a complex field, often requiring a multifaceted approach. Conventional pain treatments have long been the cornerstone of managing discomfort. These treatments typically involve the use of medications such as NSAIDs (nonsteroidal anti-inflammatory drugs) and opioids. NSAIDs, like ibuprofen and naproxen, are commonly used to reduce inflammation and alleviate pain. They work by inhibiting enzymes that contribute to inflammation, offering relief for conditions like arthritis and minor injuries. On the other hand, opioids are prescribed for more severe pain, acting on the nervous system to block pain signals to the brain. While effective, opioids come with significant risks, including the potential for dependency and a host of side effects ranging from drowsiness to gastrointestinal issues.

Beyond pharmaceuticals, physical therapy and surgical options are often considered for pain management. Physical therapy aims to improve strength and flexibility, providing long-term solutions by addressing the root cause of pain. Through targeted exercises, patients can enhance their mobility and reduce discomfort. Surgery, however, is usually reserved for cases where other treatments have failed. It can relieve structural issues but comes with recovery time and potential complications. While effective for many, these conventional methods often involve trade-offs between relief and side effects or invasive procedures.

DMSO offers a distinct advantage in the realm of pain relief. One of its greatest benefits is the reduced risk of side effects compared to traditional medications. Unlike NSAIDs and opioids, DMSO is applied topically, minimizing systemic absorption and thereby reducing the likelihood of gastrointestinal or central nervous system side effects. This localized application allows it to target specific areas of pain without affecting the entire body. Additionally, DMSO's non-invasive nature makes it an attractive option for those seeking alternatives to surgery or daily medication. It offers a natural approach, tapping into the body's healing ability with minimal external intervention.

Yet, DMSO is not without its limitations. One of the challenges is the time required to see results. While some may experience relief quickly, others might need weeks of consistent application to notice significant changes. This necessitates patience and commitment, something that can be difficult when pain is persistent. Conversely, traditional treatments often promise rapid relief, making them appealing for immediate needs. However, the prolonged use of medications like opioids carries significant risks, including dependency and tolerance. Patients may need higher doses over time, increasing the potential for adverse effects.

For many, the key lies in integrating DMSO with conventional treatments. This comprehensive approach allows for both benefits, providing a balanced strategy for pain management. DMSO can be used as a complementary therapy, enhancing the effects of physical therapy by reducing inflammation and pain and making exercises more tolerable. It can also work alongside medications, potentially allowing for lower doses and reducing the risk of side effects. Consulting with healthcare providers ensures that this integration is both safe and effective. They can guide the appropriate use of DMSO, considering your specific health needs and existing treatments.

The choice between DMSO and conventional pain treatments is not always straightforward. It involves evaluating your unique circumstances, preferences, and treatment goals. By considering the benefits and limitations of each option, you can make informed decisions that align with your health objectives. As you explore these possibilities, remember that pain management is a personal journey, one that may involve a combination of approaches to achieve optimal relief. This chapter delves into how DMSO can complement traditional methods, offering a natural and effective option for those seeking alternatives. Exploring DMSO's potential continues, promising new insights into its role in health and wellness.

# 4

## ENHANCING SKIN HEALTH AND OVERCOMING SENSITIVITIES

Imagine a mirror reflecting not the passage of time but the resilience and vitality of your skin. Our skin, much like the pages of a book, tells a story—each line and contour speaking to the years lived and experiences cherished. Yet, the quest for skin that mirrors the vitality of our spirit remains. Enter DMSO, a compound that reaches beyond the surface, offering benefits that extend far beyond merely smoothing wrinkles. It invites you to explore a broader spectrum of skin health, where hydration and elasticity form the cornerstone of a vibrant complexion.

DMSO's impact on skin hydration is profound. By enhancing moisture retention, it combats the dryness that often accompanies aging. This improved hydration is not just about appearance; it's about restoring the skin's natural barrier, protecting it from environmental aggressors. As hydration improves, so does elasticity. The skin becomes more resilient, bouncing back with a youthful vigor that defies chronological age. This dual action of hydration and elasticity is the foundation of DMSO's broader benefits, promising a complexion that feels as good as it looks.

At the cellular level, DMSO acts as a facilitator, ushering nutrients directly into skin cells. This enhanced absorption ensures that vital nutrients reach where they are most needed, promoting healthy cell turnover. It's like opening the door to a nutrient-rich banquet, where your skin cells can feast on everything they need to thrive. But DMSO doesn't stop there. It stimulates the production of collagen and elastin, the proteins that provide structure and support. Imagine them as the scaffolding beneath a canvas, giving shape and firmness to the visible layers. With increased collagen and elastin, the skin's texture becomes smoother, and the tone more even, presenting a unified, radiant appearance.

Incorporating DMSO into your skincare routine is both simple and transformative. Consider blending it with your favorite moisturizers or serums. This combination leverages DMSO's penetration-enhancing properties, driving active ingredients deeper into the skin for maximum effect. Imagine applying it to your nighttime routine when your skin's natural repair processes are most active. DMSO works harmoniously with your body as you sleep, supporting repair and renewal. This approach transforms your nightly regimen into a powerful ally in seeking healthier skin.

Real-life testimonials illuminate the potential of DMSO in skincare. Take Sarah, whose journey with acne left behind scars that marred her confidence. After integrating DMSO into her routine, she observed reduced scarring and a more even complexion. Her experience is echoed by many who have turned to DMSO for its reparative qualities. Similarly, consider John, who faced the challenges of aging skin. With DMSO, he noticed a marked improvement in smoothness, with his skin regaining the vitality he thought lost. These stories are not just anecdotes; they are testaments to DMSO's tangible benefits, bridging the gap between desire and reality.

***Interactive Element: Reflection Section***

Reflect on your skincare goals and how DMSO might help you achieve them. Consider the following prompts:

- What are the primary skin concerns you would like to address?
- How might integrating DMSO into your routine enhance your current skincare practices?
- What changes have you noticed in your skin over the years, and how could DMSO address them?

Jot down your thoughts and revisit them as you continue to explore DMSO's potential. This reflection will serve as a personal guide, aligning your efforts with your skin health aspirations.

This chapter explored how DMSO extends beyond anti-aging, offering a holistic approach to skin health. It promises a complexion reflecting vitality and resilience through improved hydration, elasticity, and nutrient absorption. The integration of DMSO into daily routines, supported by real-life testimonials, underscores its transformative potential. As you consider this information, envision how DMSO might become a valuable component of your skincare journey, unlocking new possibilities for truly more healthy skin.

## ADDRESSING SKIN SENSITIVITY: PRECAUTIONS AND TIPS

As you explore the potential benefits of DMSO for enhancing your skin health, it's crucial to be mindful of its impact on sensitive skin. Some individuals may experience sensitivity due to the concentration levels and frequency of application. DMSO, in its pure form, is potent. When applied frequently or in high concentrations, it can sometimes lead to irritation. This reaction is common and stems from the compound's ability to penetrate deeply, which, while beneficial for delivering nutrients, can also disrupt the skin's natural balance if not managed properly. Understanding your skin's unique characteristics is key. For those with sensitive skin, even the most benign substances can sometimes mean trouble, and DMSO, with its powerful properties, is no exception.

To mitigate potential adverse reactions, gradually introduce DMSO into your skincare routine. Start by applying a small amount to less reactive areas, allowing your skin to adjust to its presence. This methodical approach gives your skin time to acclimate, reducing the likelihood of irritation. Opting for lower concentrations is also a wise strategy, especially for sensitive areas like the face or neck. A diluted solution can soften DMSO's intensity, making it more gentle on the skin. By easing into the use of DMSO, you're giving your skin the chance to embrace its benefits without overwhelming it. This gradual process is akin to slowly introducing a new exercise regimen to your body, allowing time to adapt and strengthen.

Before committing to regular use, performing a patch test is a simple yet effective precaution. Choose a small, inconspicuous area of skin, such as the inside of your forearm. Apply a diluted solution of DMSO and observe the area over 24 hours. This test will reveal any immediate adverse reactions, such as redness or itching, indicating that your skin may not tolerate the compound well. If you notice any discomfort, it's a clear sign to reassess the concentration or application method. This step is essential in ensuring that you proceed safely. It's like testing a new recipe before serving it to guests, ensuring everything is just right before going all in.

ENHANCING SKIN HEALTH AND OVERCOMING SENSITIVITI... | 49

When selecting DMSO products, especially if you have sensitive skin, quality is paramount. Opt for pharmaceutical-grade DMSO, which is rigorously tested to ensure purity and safety. This grade reduces the risk of contamination, offering a cleaner, more reliable product. Additionally, steer clear of products that contain added fragrances or irritants. These additives can exacerbate sensitivity and negate the benefits of DMSO. Reading labels carefully and choosing formulations specifically designed for sensitive skin can make a world of difference. It's about making informed choices, much like selecting organic produce at the market, knowing that you're choosing the best for your health.

Navigating the world of DMSO with sensitive skin doesn't have to be daunting. With careful consideration and a methodical approach, you can unlock its potential while safeguarding your skin's health by starting slowly, testing thoroughly, and choosing high-quality products to ensure the way for a positive experience. As you incorporate DMSO into your routine, remember that your skin's needs are unique, and honoring those needs will lead to the best results.

## DMSO FOR WOUND HEALING AND RECOVERY

Wounds, whether from a minor cut or a significant surgical procedure, are a part of life that we all encounter at some point. The body's natural response to injury is a complex process aiming to repair and restore. Yet, sometimes, this process needs a little boost. Here, DMSO is a valuable ally, aiding faster recovery by reducing inflammation and pain at wound sites. Inflammation is the body's initial response to injury, characterized by redness, heat, swelling, and pain. While necessary for healing, excessive inflammation can delay recovery and increase discomfort. DMSO helps by calming this response, easing the pain, and allowing the body to focus on tissue repair. This reduction in inflammation is not just about comfort; it's about creating an optimal environment for healing.

Beyond its anti-inflammatory properties, DMSO promotes cellular regeneration and repair. It acts on the cellular level, encouraging the proliferation of fibroblasts—cells critical for forming new tissue. By accelerating the growth of these cells, DMSO supports the body's natural repair mechanisms, ensuring that wounds heal more efficiently. This action is particularly beneficial for those dealing with chronic wounds or slow-healing injuries, where the body's usual processes might need a helping hand. DMSO's role in enhancing cellular activity makes it a powerful tool in the arsenal of wound care, providing a path to quicker recovery and reduced scarring.

Applying DMSO to wounds requires careful attention to safety and hygiene. For open wounds, diluting DMSO appropriately is crucial. A standard recommendation is to mix DMSO with distilled water, creating a gentle solution for sensitive tissues. This dilution reduces the risk of irritation while delivering DMSO's benefits effectively. Cleanliness is paramount when dealing with open wounds. Ensure that the area is thoroughly cleansed before application, and use sterile tools or applicators to prevent contamination. This step is vital, as any foreign substances introduced to the wound can impede healing and lead to infection. By maintaining sterility, you create an environment conducive to healing where DMSO can work its magic without interference.

In post-surgical recovery, DMSO shines with its ability to minimize scar formation and relieve post-operative discomfort. Surgery, while often necessary, can leave behind scars that serve as permanent reminders of the procedure. DMSO helps soften these scars, promoting a smoother, more even skin surface. Its anti-inflammatory properties also play a role in reducing swelling and discomfort, common complaints in the days following surgery. DMSO accelerates recovery and enhances the overall healing experience by addressing these issues. For many, this means returning to daily activities with greater ease and confidence, free from the limitations that post-surgical pain often imposes.

Real-life examples of successful wound healing with DMSO abound. Consider the case of an athlete who suffered a significant sports injury, leaving them sidelined and frustrated. By incorporating DMSO into their recovery routine, this individual experienced a remarkable turnaround, with the injury healing faster than anticipated. This rapid recovery not only allowed them to return to the field sooner but also restored their confidence in their body's resilience. Another testimonial comes from a patient recovering from surgery, who found that regular application of DMSO significantly reduced scarring. This individual, once apprehensive about post-surgical marks, now enjoys smoother skin and a more comfortable recovery. These stories, while anecdotal, highlight the potential of DMSO to transform the healing process, offering hope and tangible results for those willing to explore its benefits.

## NAVIGATING ALLERGIES AND SKIN REACTIONS

You must be aware of possible allergic reactions when incorporating DMSO into your skincare routine. Though DMSO offers numerous benefits, it can also cause adverse reactions in some individuals. These reactions may manifest as redness, itching, or a rash, which are typical signs of an allergy. If you notice your skin becoming more sensitive, with unusual itching or redness, it might be your body's way of saying it's not in favor of DMSO. Recognizing these symptoms early is crucial, as it allows you to address the reaction promptly and minimize discomfort. Your skin's response is a reminder that what works wonders for some may not suit everyone.

If you suspect an allergic reaction to DMSO, the first step is to cease its use immediately. This gives your skin time to recover and prevents further irritation. Rinse the affected area with cool water to help soothe any itching or redness. However, it's not enough to simply stop using DMSO. Consulting a healthcare provider is essential. They can provide personalized advice and determine whether the reaction is an allergy or possibly a sensitivity to another ingredient. A professional's guidance can help you navigate this situation safely, ensuring that your skin returns to its normal state without complications.

Exploring alternative approaches is a wise course of action for those who find DMSO unsuitable. One option is to use diluted solutions mixed with natural emollients, such as aloe vera or coconut oil. These ingredients can help mitigate irritation while delivering some of DMSO's benefits. Dilution is key here, as it reduces the concentration of DMSO, making it gentler on the skin. This approach allows you to continue reaping the rewards of DMSO's properties without the risk of adverse reactions. Additionally, natural emollients have their soothing properties, providing an added layer of comfort and hydration.

Professional guidance is invaluable when dealing with allergies or adverse reactions. Dermatologists and healthcare providers can offer insights tailored to your skin's needs. They can recommend alternative treatments or adjustments to your regimen, ensuring that you continue on your path to improved skin health without discomfort. Their expertise can also help you identify any underlying factors that may be contributing to your skin's sensitivity, providing a comprehensive approach to managing allergies.

Sometimes, they suggest performing a patch test before fully committing to a new product, preventing future reactions.

A patch test is a simple yet effective way to assess your skin's compatibility with DMSO or any new product. By applying a small amount to a discreet area, such as the inside of your arm, you can observe your skin's reaction over 24 hours. This test reveals any potential issues before they become widespread, allowing you to make informed decisions about your skincare choices. If the test area shows no signs of irritation, you can proceed with greater confidence. However, if a reaction occurs, it's a clear signal to reassess the product or concentration. This step is about taking control of your skincare, ensuring you make choices that align with your skin's unique needs.

In navigating allergies and skin reactions, the goal is to find a balance that works for you. You can continue exploring DMSO's benefits while minimizing risks by being attentive to your body's signals and seeking professional advice when needed. This journey is personal, guided by your skin's responses and your commitment to maintaining its health. As you continue to explore the possibilities of DMSO, remember that your well-being is the priority, and every decision should support that aim.

In this chapter, we've explored the nuances of using DMSO for skin health, addressing potential challenges while highlighting its transformative potential. As we look ahead to the next chapter, the focus will shift to integrating DMSO with other natural remedies, expanding its benefits beyond the skin.

# DMSO FOR ADULTS AND SENIORS
## YOUR GUIDE TO NATURAL HEALING

**Relieve Chronic Pain · Reduce Inflammation · Renew Energy**

*"The best way to find yourself is to lose yourself in the service of others."*

— MAHATMA GANDHI

When we help others, we not only brighten their lives but also bring more joy to our own. Together, we can make a difference!

Would you like to help someone—just like you—who's looking for relief from pain or wondering how to feel better every day?

My goal with *DMSO for Adults and Seniors* is to make it a helpful guide for anyone exploring the benefits of natural remedies.

But here's the thing: most people choose books based on reviews. That's where you come in!

Your review doesn't just help me—it helps someone else who's curious about DMSO but unsure where to start. By sharing your thoughts, you can make a big impact.

**Why Your Review Matters**

When you leave a review, you help:

- Someone find hope and relief from pain.
- A small business grow and give back to its community.
- An entrepreneur provide for their family.

- A reader take the first step toward a healthier, happier life.

It's easy, free, and takes just a minute, but your words could change someone's journey with DMSO forever.

**How to Leave Your Review**

1. Visit this link or scan the QR code below:
2. [https://www.amazon.com/review/review-your-purchases/?asin=BOOKASIN]
3. Share your honest thoughts. (Even one sentence is helpful!)

If you're the kind of person who loves helping others, then you're exactly who I wrote this book for. Thank you for supporting this mission and helping more people discover the power of DMSO.

With heartfelt thanks,

MT Vessel

5

# INTEGRATIVE APPROACHES: COMBINING DMSO WITH OTHER NATURAL REMEDIES

In the realm of natural healing, the fusion of remedies can often lead to surprising benefits, much like a symphony where each instrument contributes to a harmonious whole. Exploring DMSO's potential has led me to discover its powerful synergy with other natural substances, creating combinations that amplify its effects. One such pairing stands out: DMSO and castor oil, a duo that has demonstrated remarkable benefits in alleviating pain and enhancing skin health.

The combination of DMSO and castor oil is a potent ally for those seeking relief from joint pain and inflammation. Each ingredient brings its strengths to the table, working together to enhance absorption and amplify anti-inflammatory effects. DMSO, known for its ability to penetrate the skin deeply, acts as a carrier, transporting the healing properties of castor oil to where they are most needed. Castor oil, derived from the castor bean plant, is rich in ricinoleic acid, which possesses anti-inflammatory and analgesic properties. When these two substances join forces, they create a powerful tool against pain, offering a natural alternative to conventional pain relief methods.

Beyond pain relief, the blend of DMSO and castor oil promotes detoxification and lymphatic drainage. The skin, our body's largest organ, is crucial in eliminating toxins. When DMSO enhances the penetration of castor oil, it aids in stimulating the lymphatic system, supporting the body's natural detox processes. This synergy not only addresses pain but also contributes to overall well-being, providing a holistic approach to health. As lymphatic flow improves, so does circulation, bringing essential nutrients to tissues and enhancing the health of joints and skin alike.

The practical applications of this combination are diverse, extending from joint pain relief to improving skin texture and reducing scar tissue. To apply this duo effectively, start with equal parts of DMSO and castor oil. Mix them thoroughly to ensure uniformity. This mixture can be applied to affected joints, where it alleviates pain and improves mobility. For skin applications, particularly in reducing scar tissue or enhancing texture, gently massage the blend into the skin, allowing it to absorb fully. Using warmth, such as a warm compress, can further enhance absorption, maximizing the benefits of this natural remedy.

To achieve optimal results, consistency is key. Regular application, ideally once or twice daily, ensures that the healing properties of DMSO and castor oil are continually delivered to the target areas. The duration of use can vary depending on the condition being treated. For chronic pain or deep-seated scars, extended use over several weeks may be necessary to see significant improvements. As with any treatment, patience and persistence are vital. While some may experience quick relief, others might find that gradual progress is the key to lasting benefits.

# INTEGRATIVE APPROACHES: COMBINING DMSO WITH OTH... | 59

The power of this combination can be seen in the stories of those who have experienced its benefits. Consider Jane, who struggled with chronic back pain for years. Traditional treatments offered little relief, leaving her frustrated and resigned. Upon discovering the combination of DMSO and castor oil, Jane began a routine of regular application. Over time, she noticed a significant reduction in pain, allowing her to enjoy activities she had long avoided. Similarly, Tom, who battled with blemishes and uneven skin texture, found his solution in this natural duo. By incorporating it into his skincare routine, Tom observed smoother skin and reduced blemishes, boosting his confidence and comfort in his skin.

***Interactive Element: Reflection Section***

Discuss how combining DMSO and castor oil might fit your wellness routine. Consider the following questions:

- What specific health concerns are you hoping to address with this combination?
- How can you incorporate the application process into your daily schedule?
- What changes have you noticed in your health that could benefit from this synergistic approach?

Take a moment to jot down your thoughts and revisit them as you explore the benefits of DMSO and castor oil. This reflection can serve as a personalized guide, helping you tailor your approach to your unique needs and goals.

This chapter delves into the remarkable synergy between DMSO and castor oil, revealing how their combined effects can transform your approach to health and wellness. By integrating these natural remedies, you unlock a powerful tool for pain relief and skin improvement, offering a path to enhanced vitality and well-being.

## COMPLEMENTARY THERAPIES: ENHANCING DMSO'S BENEFITS

Integrating complementary therapies with DMSO can create a powerful blend that amplifies its benefits. Acupuncture, with roots deep in ancient medicine, pairs beautifully with DMSO to manage pain. This practice involves inserting thin needles into specific points on the body, stimulating nerves and muscles. It's thought to improve energy flow throughout the body, which can help with pain management. When used alongside DMSO, acupuncture can offer a holistic approach to reducing discomfort. The deep penetration of DMSO, known for its anti-inflammatory properties, works in tandem with acupuncture's ability to stimulate the body's pain-relieving mechanisms. Together, they can create a more profound effect than when used separately, each enhancing the other's strengths.

Chiropractic adjustments focus on aligning the spine and improving the function of the nervous system. Many people turn to chiropractic care to alleviate chronic pain or enhance mobility. Combining these adjustments with DMSO can support structural alignment and relieve tension. Imagine the relief of a well-aligned spine, free from the pressures that cause pain and discomfort. When applied topically before an adjustment, DMSO can help relax muscles, making it easier for chiropractors to perform their work. This preparation can lead to more effective adjustments and longer-lasting relief. By enhancing the body's structural integrity, this combination targets pain and boosts overall well-being.

Adopting a holistic approach to health, these therapies contribute to reducing stress and tension, which are often underlying causes of chronic pain and other health issues. By addressing these root causes, you can promote healing and recovery. The synergy created by combining DMSO with complementary therapies like acupuncture and chiropractic care offers a broad spectrum of benefits. This integrative approach doesn't just focus on one aspect of health but encompasses the whole person. You lay the groundwork for more profound healing by reducing tension and promoting relaxation. Your body becomes more resilient and better able to cope with stressors and challenges.

When considering these therapies, scheduling regular sessions with qualified practitioners is crucial. Consistency is key to reaping the full benefits. A skilled acupuncturist or chiropractor can guide you through the process, ensuring that each session builds on the last. Finding practitioners who understand the benefits of DMSO and are willing to integrate it into their treatments can enhance the overall experience. Combining therapies into a comprehensive health plan allows you to address multiple aspects of your health simultaneously. This multi-faceted approach can accelerate healing, offering a more comprehensive solution to health challenges. By weaving these practices into your routine, you create a robust support system for your body.

Consider the case of Maria, who had struggled with chronic neck pain for years. She found that regular chiropractic adjustments, combined with DMSO, provided relief that she couldn't achieve through either method alone. The DMSO helped relax her muscles, making the adjustments more effective and reducing her pain significantly. Another example is James, who experienced enhanced mobility through the combination of DMSO and massage therapy. A skilled massage therapist used DMSO to prepare his muscles, making the massage more effective and long-lasting. These stories highlight the transformative potential of combining DMSO with complementary therapies. They serve as a testament to the enhanced relief and improved health outcomes that can be achieved through thoughtful integration. These real-world examples demonstrate how these combinations can transform your health, offering new hope and possibilities.

As you explore the potential of complementary therapies, remember that each person's experience is unique. What works for one person may not work for another, so it's important to find the right combination that suits your needs. Consulting with healthcare professionals who understand both DMSO and these complementary therapies can provide valuable guidance. They can help tailor an approach that aligns with your health goals and personal preferences. As you embark on this journey, keep an open mind and be willing to experiment. The path to optimal health is often a winding one, filled with discoveries and insights along the way.

## ANTI-INFLAMMATORY DIETS: BOOSTING DMSO'S EFFECTIVENESS

When it comes to enhancing the effectiveness of DMSO, the role of diet should not be underestimated. Consider your body a complex orchestra, where each section must work harmoniously for optimal performance. An anti-inflammatory diet serves as the conductor, guiding this ensemble toward a symphony of health. By reducing systemic inflammation, such a diet not only complements DMSO's pain-relieving properties but also supports cellular health and regeneration. This dietary approach targets inflammation at its core, addressing it before it manifests into chronic conditions that might require more invasive interventions.

Incorporating omega-3 fatty acids and antioxidants into your diet is a foundational step in this process. Omega-3s found abundantly

# INTEGRATIVE APPROACHES: COMBINING DMSO WITH OTH... | 63

in fish like salmon and mackerel, offer powerful anti-inflammatory benefits. They help reduce inflammatory markers in the body, aligning perfectly with DMSO's properties. Antioxidants, on the other hand, are your body's defense against oxidative stress, a contributor to inflammation. Foods rich in antioxidants, such as berries, dark chocolate, and leafy greens, can bolster your body's natural defenses, working alongside DMSO to promote healing and reduce pain.

Equally important is eliminating processed foods and inflammatory triggers from your diet. These culprits, often laden with sugars and unhealthy fats, can exacerbate inflammation and counteract the benefits of DMSO. By steering clear of processed foods, you create an environment within your body that welcomes healing and rejuvenation. Instead, focus on whole, nutrient-dense foods that nourish your body and support its natural healing processes. This shift not only enhances DMSO's effectiveness but also contributes to overall health and well-being, creating a cycle of positive reinforcement.

Consider starting your day with a turmeric and ginger smoothie to assist you on this path. Both turmeric and ginger are renowned for their anti-inflammatory properties, providing a natural boost to your health regimen. Blend a teaspoon of turmeric and a slice of fresh ginger with a banana, a handful of spinach, and a cup of almond milk. This vibrant concoction tastes refreshing and sets the tone for a day focused on health and vitality. As you make this smoothie a part of your routine, you'll likely notice more than just improved energy levels; you'll feel a sense of clarity and balance throughout your day.

A weekly meal plan focused on anti-inflammatory foods can further support your health goals. Begin your week with grilled salmon alongside a quinoa salad rich in spinach and walnuts.

Midweek, consider a hearty lentil soup with vegetables like carrots and kale. Round out the week with roasted sweet potatoes and a side of sautéed Brussels sprouts seasoned with olive oil and garlic. These meals, simple yet flavorful, provide a roadmap to integrating anti-inflammatory foods into your life. As you follow this plan, you may notice a decrease in joint discomfort, making it easier to engage in activities that bring you joy.

Testimonials from those who have embraced dietary changes alongside DMSO usage provide compelling evidence of the benefits. Take, for example, the experience of Linda, who struggled with joint discomfort for years. Her joint pain significantly decreased after adopting an anti-inflammatory diet rich in omega-3s and antioxidants. Coupled with regular DMSO application, Linda reported not only improved mobility but also a newfound sense of freedom in her daily life. Her story underscores the power of combining dietary changes with DMSO, offering a holistic approach to managing inflammation and pain.

Similarly, consider the case of David, who sought to enhance his energy levels and vitality. By incorporating more whole foods and reducing his intake of processed items, he noticed a marked improvement in his overall well-being. Alongside DMSO, these dietary adjustments provided David with sustained energy throughout the day, allowing him to participate more fully in activities he loves. His experience illustrates the synergy between diet and DMSO, highlighting how dietary changes can amplify the compound's benefits, transforming not just physical health but also overall quality of life.

## YOGA AND EXERCISE: PROMOTING MOBILITY AND HEALING WITH DMSO

Integrating yoga and exercise with DMSO can significantly enhance the compound's benefits, creating a powerful alliance for health and mobility. Physical activity, particularly yoga, is pivotal in improving flexibility and muscle strength, often compromised by aging or chronic conditions. Yoga's gentle stretches and poses help lengthen muscles, increasing range of motion and reducing stiffness. This complements DMSO's ability to penetrate deeply and alleviate pain, creating a dual approach that addresses symptoms and underlying causes of immobility. As muscles strengthen and joints become more flexible, everyday movements become easier, enhancing your quality of life. This synergy is particularly effective for individuals with joint pain or stiffness, as the combination of yoga and DMSO fosters a more comfortable and active lifestyle.

Furthermore, incorporating regular exercise supports cardiovascular health and circulation, two critical factors in maintaining overall well-being. Exercise promotes healthy blood flow, ensuring that oxygen and nutrients reach all body parts, including those affected by inflammation or injury. When DMSO is used alongside exercise, it can enhance these benefits by reducing inflammation and pain, making physical activity more accessible and less daunting. Improved circulation also aids in the elimination of toxins, supporting the body's natural detoxification processes. This holistic approach not only targets physical symptoms but also encourages a healthier, more vibrant life by promoting cardiovascular fitness.

For those looking to incorporate specific exercises that complement DMSO, certain yoga poses can be particularly beneficial. Poses such as the cat-cow stretch and child's pose gently stretch the spine and relieve tension, making them ideal for reducing joint stiffness. These poses can be performed daily, integrating seamlessly into your routine. They not only improve flexibility but also promote relaxation, reducing stress and tension that can exacerbate pain. Strength training exercises, such as leg presses or seated rows, can also support joint health by building muscle strength around the joints. This added support can alleviate joint pressure, reducing pain and enhancing mobility.

Consistency and gradual progression are paramount when combining exercise with DMSO use. Start with gentle exercises to give your body time to adjust, and gradually increase intensity as your strength and flexibility improve. This approach prevents overexertion and reduces the risk of injury, allowing you to build a sustainable exercise routine that supports long-term health. Consistency ensures that the benefits of both exercise and DMSO are realized, as regular activity reinforces the improvements gained from the DMSO application. This balanced strategy fosters a healthier lifestyle, encouraging you to move more freely and confidently.

The transformative power of combining DMSO with exercise is best illustrated through real-life success stories. Consider the experience of Anne, a senior who had long struggled with limited mobility due to arthritis. Anne gradually regained her independence by integrating gentle yoga practices with DMSO applications. She found that her morning yoga routine and DMSO helped alleviate stiffness and pain, allowing her to enjoy activities she once thought impossible. Similarly, Tom, an athlete recovering from a sports injury, discovered enhanced recovery and performance through this combination. DMSO helped reduce inflammation, while targeted exercises strengthened his muscles and accelerated healing. Tom's story is a testament to the powerful synergy between DMSO and exercise, showcasing how this partnership can improve health outcomes and renewed vitality.

6

# OVERCOMING SKEPTICISM: THE EVIDENCE FOR DMSO

Imagine standing at a crossroads, where one path leads to the comfort of traditional treatments while the other invites you to explore new possibilities with DMSO. This juncture is where many find themselves grappling with skepticism and uncertainty. DMSO, a compound with a rich history, offers intriguing benefits, yet it is often shrouded in doubt. Understanding the roots of this skepticism is crucial to moving forward. Historically, DMSO has been a subject of controversy. Developed in the 19th century, its journey from chemical solvent to medical marvel has been challenging. Early studies sparked excitement but also led to exaggerated claims, creating a landscape where skepticism could thrive. Concerns about efficacy and safety lingered, fueled by misinformation and a lack of clear scientific consensus.

People often voice fears about DMSO, focusing on potential side effects and unknown long-term impacts. These concerns are not unfounded. While DMSO is generally safe when used correctly, reports of skin irritation, gastrointestinal discomfort, and a garlic-like odor have raised eyebrows. The worry over these side effects is compounded by a broader fear of the unknown. Without extensive long-term studies, some see DMSO as a gamble. This apprehension is exacerbated by the anecdotal nature of much evidence supporting DMSO. While personal stories of relief and recovery are compelling, they lack the rigorous validation of controlled clinical trials. Critics argue that these accounts, while hopeful, do not provide a comprehensive picture of DMSO's capabilities and limitations.

To address and mitigate this skepticism, education has become a powerful tool. By equipping ourselves with knowledge, we can approach DMSO with confidence. Encouraging informed decision-making starts with accessing reliable resources and research. Look for studies published in reputable journals, and consult healthcare professionals who understand the nuances of DMSO. These experts can offer insights grounded in both science and practical experience, helping to dispel myths and misconceptions. Additionally, providing clear information about proper usage and potential side effects allows individuals to weigh the benefits and risks thoughtfully. This transparency fosters trust and empowers you to make choices aligned with your health goals.

Open-mindedness is paramount when exploring alternative treatments like DMSO. Approaching this compound with curiosity rather than skepticism can open doors to new possibilities. It's important to weigh the pros and cons, recognizing that every treatment has strengths and limitations. A balanced perspective involves acknowledging both the potential benefits and the challenges. This mindset encourages a trial-based approach, where you can explore DMSO's effects under supervision, adjusting as needed. By treating it as a complementary tool rather than a cure-all, you create a space for DMSO to support your wellness journey harmoniously.

***Reflection Section: Exploring Your Skepticism***

Consider the following questions as you reflect on your feelings about DMSO:

- What specific concerns or doubts do you have about DMSO?
- How might learning more about DMSO's history and scientific research address these concerns?
- Are there experiences with alternative treatments that influence your perception of DMSO?

Jot down your thoughts and revisit them as you continue to explore the potential of DMSO. This reflection will serve as a guide, helping you navigate your skepticism with clarity and openness.

In navigating skepticism, remember that it is a natural part of exploring new health options. By grounding your understanding in research and maintaining an open mind, you can make informed decisions that best support your health and well-being. The path forward involves curiosity and a willingness to explore the potential of DMSO, armed with both knowledge and a balanced perspective.

## SCIENTIFIC STUDIES: WHAT THE RESEARCH SAYS ABOUT DMSO

The scientific exploration of DMSO spans decades, with numerous studies investigating its potential benefits and applications. One of the most compelling aspects of DMSO is its role in pain relief. Randomized controlled trials have shown promising results, particularly in alleviating conditions like osteoarthritis and rheumatoid arthritis. These studies often focus on DMSO's ability to reduce joint pain and improve function, comparing its effects to standard treatments. The findings suggest that DMSO can provide significant relief, making it a viable option for those seeking alternatives to traditional pain medications. In some trials, participants reported decreased pain levels and increased mobility, highlighting DMSO's potential to improve the quality of life for individuals with chronic pain conditions.

Beyond pain relief, meta-analyses have explored DMSO's anti-inflammatory effects, compiling data from various studies to assess its overall efficacy. These analyses reveal that DMSO's anti-inflammatory properties are not only consistent but also significant across different conditions. By reducing the production of inflammatory cytokines, DMSO helps mitigate the body's inflammatory response. This ability to lower inflammation is particularly beneficial for individuals with autoimmune diseases or chronic inflammatory conditions. The meta-analyses underscore DMSO's role as an effective anti-inflammatory agent, reinforcing its potential as a therapeutic tool. Despite these promising findings, it's crucial to consider the limitations of the existing research.

The credibility of DMSO studies varies, with factors like sample size and study duration influencing their reliability. Some studies involve small sample sizes, which can limit the generalizability of the results. Larger studies are needed to confirm the findings and provide a more comprehensive understanding of DMSO's effects. Study duration also plays a role, as short-term trials may not capture the long-term impact of DMSO use. Potential biases and conflicts of interest can further complicate the picture. Researchers with ties to DMSO manufacturers may unconsciously skew results favoring the compound. It's essential to approach the research critically, recognizing these limitations while appreciating its insights.

Recent advancements in DMSO research have opened new avenues for its application. In dermatology, innovative uses of DMSO have emerged thanks to its ability to enhance the penetration of therapeutic agents. This property makes DMSO a valuable tool in treating conditions like scleroderma and ischemic ulcers. Researchers are also exploring its potential in neurological conditions, where DMSO's anti-inflammatory and neuroprotective effects could prove beneficial. Early studies indicate that DMSO may help reduce brain swelling and improve outcomes in traumatic brain injury patients. These breakthroughs highlight the versatility of DMSO and its potential to address a wide range of health challenges.

A wealth of resources is available for those interested in delving deeper into the world of DMSO research. Peer-reviewed journals like "The Journal of Rheumatology" and "The International Journal of Dermatology" frequently publish studies on DMSO, offering valuable insights into its applications and effects. Books such as "DMSO: Nature's Healer" by Dr. Morton Walker provide a comprehensive overview of DMSO's history and uses. Expert interviews with researchers and practitioners can also shed light on the nuances of the DMSO application. These resources serve as a starting point for those eager to expand their understanding and explore the potential of DMSO further.

In navigating the landscape of DMSO research, it's important to remember that science is ever-evolving. New studies and discoveries continue to shape our understanding of this compound, revealing both its potential and limitations. By staying informed and critically evaluating the research, you can make educated decisions about incorporating DMSO into your health regimen. The journey of discovery never truly ends, as each study adds a new piece to the puzzle, enhancing our grasp of DMSO's place in the realm of natural therapies.

## ADDRESSING CONCERNS: SAFETY AND EFFICACY OF DMSO

When considering the use of DMSO, understanding its safety profile is paramount. The FDA has approved DMSO for specific medical applications, notably for treating interstitial cystitis, a painful bladder condition. This approval underscores its recognized safety when used under medical guidance. Yet, like any compound, DMSO is not without its side effects. Common reactions include skin irritation and a garlic-like odor on the breath, a benign, albeit sometimes unwelcome, side effect due to its sulfur content. These effects are typically mild and manageable, often subsiding as your body adjusts. Ensuring you use pharmaceutical-grade DMSO rather than industrial-grade is crucial, as the latter may contain impurities harmful when absorbed through the skin. It's wise to start with a patch test, applying DMSO to a small area to monitor your skin's reaction. This test is a straightforward way to avoid broader adverse effects, offering peace of mind as you integrate DMSO into your routine.

Efficacy is where DMSO truly shines, supported by a wealth of scientific evidence that highlights its benefits across various conditions. In the realm of pain management, DMSO has demonstrated significant efficacy. Clinical trials have shown that it can reduce pain and inflammation, particularly in conditions like arthritis, where its anti-inflammatory properties are most beneficial. Participants often report not only a decrease in pain but also improved mobility, which can significantly enhance quality of life. Beyond arthritis, DMSO is used in dermatology for its ability to enhance the penetration of other therapeutic agents, making it highly effective in treating skin conditions such as scleroderma and ischemic ulcers. These applications reflect DMSO's versatility and its potential to address a wide array of health concerns. The evidence for DMSO is in controlled studies, and the voices of countless users who have experienced its benefits firsthand offer a practical perspective on its efficacy.

To maximize the benefits of DMSO while minimizing risks, it is crucial to follow recommended dosages and applications. Start with a lower concentration, typically around 70%, and gradually increase as needed, monitoring your body's response. The dosage depends on the treated condition, with topical application being the most common method. Applying DMSO to clean skin ensures better absorption and reduces the risk of irritation. It's important to apply DMSO cautiously, avoiding sensitive areas like the eyes and mucous membranes. Monitoring for adverse reactions is essential. If you notice any unusual symptoms, such as severe irritation or allergic reactions, discontinue use and consult a healthcare professional. They can provide personalized advice and suggest alternative approaches if necessary. Consulting with a healthcare provider before starting DMSO, especially if you are on other medications, can prevent potential interactions and ensure safe use.

One common concern among skeptics is the perceived toxicity of DMSO. This concern often stems from misunderstandings about its chemical nature and history as an industrial solvent. However, DMSO is safe for medical use when used correctly, as evidenced by its FDA approval. Its toxicity is low when compared to many pharmaceuticals, and it is generally well-tolerated by most individuals. Long-term safety is another area where evidence supports DMSO's use. Studies have shown that, when used appropriately, DMSO does not lead to significant long-term adverse effects. This reassurance is backed by decades of research and clinical use, offering confidence to those hesitant to try this compound.

Understanding these facts can help dispel myths and provide a clearer picture of what DMSO can offer.

For those deciding to use DMSO, it's essential to weigh the evidence and approach it with informed confidence. The path to integrating DMSO into your health regimen involves understanding its safety, acknowledging its benefits, and using it responsibly. This approach ensures that you harness its potential effectively, paving the way for improved health outcomes.

## BUSTING THE "TOO GOOD TO BE TRUE" MYTH

The allure of DMSO often lies in its portrayal as a wonder compound capable of addressing a myriad of health issues with ease. This perception, however, deserves a closer look. Many people label DMSO as "too good to be true," and it's essential to understand why. Misleading marketing and exaggerated testimonials play a significant role in shaping this view. Advertisements and anecdotal stories sometimes paint DMSO as a miracle solution without acknowledging its complexities and nuances. This portrayal can lead to unrealistic expectations, creating disappointment when the compound doesn't deliver instant or miraculous results. Furthermore, a lack of awareness about the scientific basis of DMSO contributes to this myth. Without a solid understanding of how DMSO works and its limitations, it's easy to fall for the hype and overlook its genuine benefits.

To provide a balanced perspective, it's crucial to differentiate between the realistic benefits of DMSO and the overhyped claims that often surround it. Setting realistic expectations is key for new users. DMSO is not a cure-all, but it can be a valuable tool for managing specific conditions. Its effectiveness depends on various factors, including the particular health issue being addressed and how it's applied. For example, while DMSO can reduce inflammation and improve joint mobility, it may not eliminate pain or replace other treatments. Understanding these limitations helps users appreciate what DMSO can genuinely offer without falling into the trap of thinking it can solve all health problems. By focusing on its proven capabilities, users can make informed decisions and use DMSO effectively as part of a broader wellness strategy.

Case studies and expert opinions provide valuable insights into DMSO's practical applications, helping dispel the myths surrounding it. One case study highlights the long-term benefits of DMSO without resorting to miraculous claims. A patient with chronic arthritis used DMSO consistently over several months, experiencing gradual improvement in joint flexibility and a reduction in pain. This steady progress showcases DMSO's potential when used appropriately and with patience. Expert commentary further reinforces these findings, emphasizing that DMSO's true strength lies in its ability to complement existing treatments rather than replace them. Professionals in the field often note that while DMSO can enhance the effects of other therapies, it should be used as part of a comprehensive health plan tailored to individual needs.

Encouraging critical thinking and personal experimentation is essential for those exploring DMSO. Users can approach DMSO with curiosity and caution by adopting an open yet analytical mindset. Documenting personal experiences with DMSO can provide valuable insights into its effects and help identify the most effective ways to use it. This practice allows users to track symptom changes and adjust their approach as needed, ensuring that DMSO is used safely and effectively. Balancing optimism with evidence-based caution is another crucial aspect of using DMSO wisely. While hoping for positive outcomes is natural, it's essential to remain grounded in reality and base decisions on credible information. This balanced approach empowers users to explore DMSO's potential while remaining mindful of its limitations.

As we draw this chapter to a close, exploring DMSO's potential continues, promising new insights into its role in health and wellness.

# 7

# FINANCIAL ACCESSIBILITY AND QUALITY ASSURANCE

In the realm of natural healing, cost can often be a barrier to accessing the remedies that promise relief. When I first discovered DMSO, my primary concern was its effectiveness and how to make it an affordable part of my health regimen. The balance between quality and cost is delicate, yet it is essential to ensure that these treatments remain accessible to all who need them. In this chapter, we explore how to navigate the financial aspects of DMSO, offering practical solutions that make this powerful compound attainable without straining your budget.

## COST-EFFECTIVE SOLUTIONS: MAKING DMSO AFFORDABLE

Finding DMSO at a reasonable price starts with understanding the landscape of purchasing options. Bulk purchasing stands out as one of the most effective strategies for cost savings. Buying in larger quantities often reduces the price per unit, making it a smart choice for long-term users. Many suppliers, like those on websites such as Covalent Chemical, offer DMSO in bulk, allowing you to purchase enough to last several months. This approach lowers costs and ensures you always have a supply on hand, reducing reordering frequency. It's akin to stocking up on pantry essentials, ensuring that you never run out of what you need most.

Discounts and promotions are another avenue to explore when seeking affordable DMSO. Many reputable suppliers offer seasonal sales or discounts for first-time buyers. Keeping an eye on these opportunities can lead to significant savings. Subscribe to newsletters from trusted suppliers or set alerts on e-commerce platforms to catch these deals as they arise. It's like shopping for holiday presents during sales events, where a little patience and timing can lead to substantial financial relief.

Pooling resources with others is a powerful strategy that leverages community and shared interests. Organizing group purchases with friends or local health groups can drastically cut costs. By buying together, each participant can benefit from bulk pricing without storing large quantities individually. This communal approach not only saves money but also fosters a sense of connection and shared purpose. Online forums and social media groups dedicated to natural health can be excellent places to find others interested in group buying. These platforms serve as modern marketplaces where like-minded individuals come together to support one another.

Comparing prices across different vendors is crucial for ensuring you get the best deal. Price comparison tools and websites are invaluable resources in this endeavor. These platforms allow you to instantly enter the product you seek and compare prices from multiple suppliers. This transparency empowers you to make informed decisions, ensuring that you don't pay more than necessary. It's the digital equivalent of shopping around town without the hassle of visiting multiple stores. By utilizing these tools, you can pinpoint the most cost-effective sources for DMSO, aligning your purchase with your financial goals.

Reducing overall treatment costs with DMSO also involves strategic use and combination with other remedies. By integrating DMSO with cost-effective natural remedies, you enhance its benefits while minimizing expenses. For example, combining DMSO with essential oils, which are known for their complementary pain relief and anti-inflammatory properties, can amplify results. This synergy allows you to reduce the amount of DMSO needed per application, stretching your supply further. Another practical tip is to minimize waste by using precise application techniques. Instead of applying DMSO liberally, use a measured approach, focusing only on the affected areas. This precision conserves the product and ensures that each application is as effective as possible.

*Interactive Element: Cost-Saving Checklist*

To help manage your DMSO-related expenses, consider this checklist:

- **Bulk Purchasing**: Identify suppliers offering bulk options and calculate potential savings.
- **Discount Alerts**: Subscribe to newsletters from reputable suppliers for promotions.
- **Community Buying**: Connect with local groups or online forums interested in group purchases.
- **Price Comparison**: Use online tools to compare prices across multiple vendors.
- **Efficient Use**: Combine DMSO with other remedies and apply carefully to avoid waste.

This checklist serves as a guide to navigating the financial aspects of using DMSO, ensuring that you can access its benefits without compromising your budget. By adopting these strategies, you can integrate DMSO into your wellness routine in a way that is both sustainable and economical.

## CHOOSING HIGH-QUALITY DMSO PRODUCTS

When considering the addition of DMSO to your health regimen, ensuring the quality of the product you purchase is crucial. The marketplace is vast, and not all DMSO products are created equal. To start, focus on purity levels and concentration specifics. High-quality DMSO should have a purity level of at least 99.9%, ensuring that your application is free from impurities that could compromise its effectiveness or safety. This purity level is a hallmark of pharmaceutical-grade DMSO, a certification that indicates it meets rigorous standards for use in medical applications. Such certifications not only guarantee purity but also consistency in concentration, which is essential for achieving reliable results with each use.

Reputable suppliers play a pivotal role in quality assurance. Selecting a trusted vendor can mean the difference between receiving a product that genuinely benefits your health and falling short. Start by researching supplier reviews and testimonials. These firsthand accounts can provide valuable insights into the experiences of other customers, helping you gauge the reliability and reputability of a supplier. Additionally, ensure that the supplier complies with safety standards and regulations. This compliance is a safeguard, ensuring that their products are tested and verified for safe use. A reputable supplier will often provide detailed product information, including certificates of analysis, which further confirm the authenticity and quality of their DMSO.

Verifying product authenticity is another critical step. Begin by examining the packaging and labeling for authenticity markers. High-quality DMSO products should have clear and professional labeling that includes essential details such as the batch number and production date. These details not only confirm that the product is genuine but also that it is fresh and has not been sitting on a shelf for an extended period. The presence of a batch number is particularly important, as it allows you to trace the product back to its source, ensuring full transparency from production to purchase. Authentic products will also feature tamper-evident seals, a simple yet effective way to guarantee that your purchase has not been compromised.

The risks associated with using low-quality or counterfeit DMSO should not be underestimated. Products not meeting high purity standards can increase skin irritation risks and adverse reactions. When impurities are present, they can provoke unexpected responses, undermining the therapeutic benefits of DMSO and potentially causing harm. Beyond irritation, the effectiveness of your treatment could be compromised. Low-quality DMSO may not deliver the intended results, leading to frustration and a lack of progress in your health goals. This potential for ineffectiveness underscores the importance of choosing high-quality products from the outset. By doing so, you ensure that each application of DMSO contributes positively to your well-being.

In summary, selecting high-quality DMSO involves carefully balancing research, verification, and trust. By prioritizing purity levels and reputable suppliers, you lay the foundation for a successful and safe experience with DMSO. Whether you're using it for pain relief, inflammation reduction, or skin health, the quality of the product directly influences the outcomes you achieve. Take the time to verify authenticity and avoid the pitfalls of low-quality alternatives, ensuring that your investment in DMSO translates into tangible benefits for your health. Through diligence and informed choices, you can navigate the market with confidence, securing a product that aligns with your wellness objectives.

## COMPARING COSTS: DMSO VS. TRADITIONAL TREATMENTS

When evaluating the financial aspects of DMSO against conventional treatments, the potential for long-term savings becomes a compelling advantage. In contrast to pharmaceuticals, which often require ongoing purchases and can accumulate significant expenses over time, DMSO presents a more sustainable financial picture. While there is an initial investment, particularly if purchasing in bulk, the cost per use is comparatively lower. Consider the routine prescriptions many endure—each refill represents another expense, often compounded by the necessity of additional medications to manage side effects. With DMSO, its relief frequently reduces the need for supplementary drugs, translating to tangible savings not just monetarily but in overall health management. This long-term perspective, where the upfront costs of DMSO are offset by reduced dependency on expensive pharmaceuticals, offers a financially sound alternative for many seeking relief from chronic conditions.

The hidden costs associated with traditional treatments extend beyond the pharmacy counter. Often, these treatments necessitate frequent doctor visits to manage the primary condition and monitor and adjust medication dosages. Each visit carries its own costs—co-pays, transportation, and time away from other activities. Additionally, the side effects of many conventional medications may require further prescriptions, adding layers of expense. For instance, a medication prescribed for arthritis pain may lead to gastrointestinal issues, necessitating additional drugs to counteract these effects. This cycle can create an overwhelming financial burden, where the true cost of treatment is not just in the medication itself but in the cascading expenses it generates. DMSO minimizes these hidden costs by potentially alleviating chronic pain and inflammation more naturally, simplifying the overall treatment landscape.

The financial benefits of DMSO have been vividly illustrated through the experiences of individuals who have shifted away from traditional medications. Take, for instance, the story of a woman who, after years of managing her arthritis with prescriptions, turned to DMSO. Through diligent application and integration into her routine, she found she could significantly reduce her reliance on expensive arthritis medications. This shift led not only to monetary savings but also to an improved quality of life, free from the side effects that plagued her with previous treatments. Her story is a testament to the economic viability of DMSO, highlighting how one can achieve relief without the financial strain often associated with chronic illness management. Similarly, a case study involving a man with chronic back pain demonstrated a notable decrease in healthcare expenses. By adopting a holistic approach that included DMSO, he was able to cut down on physical therapy sessions and prescription costs, further underscoring DMSO's potential to streamline and economize health care.

Determining personal savings when transitioning to DMSO from traditional medications can be facilitated by practical tools designed for this very purpose. Budget planners and cost-comparison spreadsheets allow you to meticulously track expenses, clearly showing your financial commitments. You can visualize potential savings by inputting the costs of traditional treatments and comparing them against the expenses associated with DMSO. These tools also help identify areas where you might optimize your spending, ensuring that every dollar contributes effectively to your health goals. Online calculators for medication cost analysis further simplify this process. By entering specific details about your current prescriptions, these calculators can project potential savings when switching to or integrating DMSO. They provide a straightforward way to assess the financial impact of your health choices, empowering you to make informed decisions that align with both your health and financial objectives.

For many, the decision to incorporate DMSO into their health regimen is driven by the promise of reduced expenses and improved well-being. The shift eases financial burdens and simplifies the complexity of managing chronic conditions. As you weigh the costs and benefits of DMSO against traditional treatments, consider the broader implications—less frequent doctor visits, fewer side effects, and the liberation from dependency on multiple medications. This perspective underscores DMSO's potential to transform both health and financial landscapes, offering a viable path toward sustainable wellness.

### DIY HEALTH PRACTICES: ECONOMICAL USE OF DMSO

Taking control of your health often involves a hands-on approach, and creating your DMSO-based solutions can significantly enhance both your treatment's effectiveness and affordability. By blending DMSO with essential oils, you can tailor your applications to meet specific needs, whether it's soothing inflammation or enhancing skin health. Essential oils like lavender, peppermint, or eucalyptus complement DMSO's properties and add their therapeutic benefits. Imagine crafting a personalized blend that targets your unique health concerns, offering both physical relief and the pleasing aroma of natural oils. This personalization makes your treatment more enjoyable and ensures you use ingredients you're comfortable with, avoiding unwanted additives or chemicals in some commercial products.

Creating personalized treatment regimens at home doesn't have to be daunting. Start by gathering your supplies: a high-quality bottle of DMSO, your chosen essential oils, and a carrier oil such as coconut or jojoba oil. A carrier oil acts as a base, ensuring the DMSO and essential oils blend smoothly for application. Begin by measuring a small amount of DMSO and combining it with the carrier oil, typically in a 1:1 ratio, although you can adjust this based on your skin's sensitivity and the concentration you desire. Add a few drops of essential oil to this mixture, stirring gently to blend. Once mixed, store your homemade blend in a glass container to preserve its integrity. This method not only stretches the use of DMSO but also customizes the treatment to your specific needs, allowing you to focus on areas requiring the most attention.

The benefits of do-it-yourself practices extend beyond mere cost savings. Customization is perhaps the most significant advantage, as it allows you to cater to your individual health needs. Each body is different, and a one-size-fits-all approach rarely yields the best results. Creating your blends will enable you to adjust the concentration and ingredients to suit your health goals. Additionally, this hands-on involvement fosters a more in-depth understanding of what works for your body, encouraging a proactive stance on health management. This empowerment can be transformative, providing not only physical relief but also a sense of independence and confidence in your ability to manage your health.

The potential of DIY health practices lies in their ability to transform how you approach treatment. By actively participating in creating your remedies, you gain valuable insights into the ingredients and processes that best support your health. This knowledge empowers you to refine your methods over time, ensuring that your treatments evolve to meet changing needs. Furthermore, it fosters a deeper connection to your health journey, where you are not just a passive recipient of care but an active participant in shaping your path to wellness. This engagement can lead to more sustainable health practices focusing on long-term well-being rather than short-term fixes.

As we close this chapter, we've seen how DIY practices with DMSO offer more than just economical solutions—they provide a personalized approach to health that can be as rewarding as it is effective. This exploration of self-crafted treatments highlights the power of tailoring remedies to individual needs, bridging the gap between cost and care. These methods remind us of the potential within our reach when we combine knowledge with action. As we look ahead, the focus will shift to building supportive communities and connections, enhancing our understanding and use of DMSO in everyday life.

# 8

## COMMUNITY AND SUPPORT: BUILDING CONNECTIONS

Imagine a circle of friends gathered around a table, each sharing their latest experiences and insights into health and wellness. This lively exchange is more than just conversation; it's a lifeline, offering support and encouragement. In today's connected world, these circles have expanded beyond physical spaces, reaching into the vast expanse of the internet. Online forums and local groups are vibrant communities where knowledge flows freely, and support is just a click away. These platforms are crucial for anyone exploring new health avenues, such as DMSO. They provide a space where you can ask questions, share experiences, and find the collective wisdom of those who have walked similar paths.

Online forums are particularly valuable, offering various experiences and advice. They bring together individuals from different backgrounds, each contributing their unique perspectives. This diversity enriches discussions and broadens your understanding, presenting a tapestry of insights that might be challenging to find elsewhere. You can pose questions anonymously in these virtual spaces, allowing for honest and open dialogue. Whether you're curious about the best DMSO applications or seeking advice on managing potential side effects, forums provide a supportive environment to explore these topics.

Finding the right online community can be daunting. Start by evaluating the credibility of forum moderators and contributors. Look for platforms with knowledgeable moderators who ensure that discussions remain respectful and informative. It's also essential to check for forum rules and community guidelines. Reputable forums will have clear standards that promote constructive interactions and protect members from misinformation. Platforms like the *Forum for Integrative Medicine* offer a good example of such communities, where professional input complements user experiences, fostering a well-rounded discussion environment.

While online forums offer convenience, local support groups provide a tangible connection that can be deeply rewarding. In-person meetings allow you to build personal connections and friendships, offering a sense of camaraderie that is sometimes missing online. These gatherings provide an opportunity to engage directly with others who are experimenting with or using DMSO. You can share your stories, learn from others, and even witness the transformation of fellow members. Participating in local health and wellness events organized by these groups can also enhance your understanding and application of DMSO.

Starting or joining a local group requires initiative but can be incredibly fulfilling. Use social media to organize local meetups. Platforms like Facebook or Meetup.com are excellent tools for finding like-minded individuals in your area. You can create events, invite members, and coordinate meetings with ease. Collaboration is key to building a successful group. Partner with local wellness centers or libraries, as resources and spaces are often available for community gatherings. These venues can host events, workshops, or regular meetings, providing a consistent place for members to gather and share ideas. By fostering these local connections, you contribute to a network of support that can significantly enhance your health journey.

*Interactive Element: Finding Your Community*

- **Checklist for Evaluating Online Forums:**
    - Verify moderator credentials and activity.
    - Review community guidelines for respectful engagement.
    - Look for a diverse range of topics and active discussions.
- **Tips for starting a Local Group:**
    - Use social media to gauge interest and organize meetings.
    - Partner with local wellness centers for resources and venues.
    - Schedule regular meetings to maintain engagement and momentum.

Whether you find support online or in person, these communities can be a cornerstone of your health exploration. They offer a wealth of knowledge and a network of encouragement, helping you navigate the complexities of using DMSO. Through these connections, you're not alone; you're part of a larger tapestry of individuals striving for better health and well-being. Be sure to check out the reference and links pages at the end of the book.

## SHARING EXPERIENCES: TESTIMONIALS AND TIPS

Stories have an incredible power to inspire and educate, especially those who have faced similar challenges. Personal testimonials are not just tales of individual journeys; they are beacons of hope and reservoirs of practical wisdom. When someone shares their success with DMSO, it lights a path for others navigating similar health struggles. These stories provide motivation, reminding us that change is possible and that others have walked this road before and found relief. Real-life experiences often bring to light practical tips that might not be covered in medical literature. They offer insights into what worked and what didn't and the subtle nuances that can significantly affect treatment outcomes.

Encouraging readers to share their journeys is vital in fostering a thriving community. By contributing their stories, individuals add to the collective knowledge pool, enriching the community with diverse perspectives. Writing blog posts or articles for community websites is one way to broadcast these experiences. Such platforms often reach a wide audience, spreading valuable information and potentially helping someone who feels isolated in their struggle. Participation in discussion panels or webinars also offers a dynamic way to share insights. These interactive sessions allow for real-time exchange of ideas and can spark new approaches to using DMSO effectively.

The beauty of community lies in its reciprocal nature. The act of giving and receiving feedback creates a cycle of continuous learning and support. When you share your experiences, others gain from your insights, just as you learn from theirs. This exchange enriches everyone involved, providing a broader understanding of DMSO's potential. Learning from others' successes can offer new strategies, while their challenges highlight pitfalls to avoid. Adapting a personal plan based on peer feedback refines your approach and fosters a sense of belonging and shared purpose. This dynamic interaction makes the community a living entity, continually evolving and adapting to new information and experiences.

Examples of impactful testimonials illustrate this beautifully. One story that resonates is of an individual who initially approached DMSO with skepticism. Through community encouragement, they decided to give it a try and subsequently found significant relief from chronic pain. Their journey from doubt to healing inspired others to reconsider and provided practical insights into managing dosage and application techniques. Another story involves a community member discovering new applications for DMSO through shared experiences. By learning about others' successes with DMSO in skincare, they ventured into using it for similar issues and found unexpected benefits. These stories highlight the transformative power of sharing and the endless possibilities that can emerge from a supportive network of peers.

## COMMUNITY WORKSHOPS: LEARNING AND GROWING TOGETHER

Workshops serve as a dynamic engine for community building, creating a space where learning transcends individual boundaries and becomes a shared endeavor. They offer hands-on experience with DMSO applications, allowing participants to see and feel the processes firsthand, which can be far more illuminating than reading or watching videos. Imagine working alongside others, trying application techniques, and discussing immediate results. This tactile engagement fosters a deeper understanding and often leads to those "aha" moments that are so crucial in health exploration. Expert-led sessions also elevate these gatherings, introducing advanced topics that might seem daunting on your own.

Having a knowledgeable guide to navigate these complexities can make all the difference, providing insights into DMSO that you might not encounter elsewhere. These experts can address nuanced questions and suggest new angles for consideration, broadening your understanding of DMSO's potential.

Organizing or participating in these workshops requires some planning but is immensely rewarding. Collaboration is key. Partnering with healthcare professionals for workshop leadership not only lends credibility to the event but also ensures that the information shared is accurate and beneficial. These professionals can bring their clinical expertise, offering guidance that is both practical and scientifically grounded. It's essential to set clear objectives and agendas for each session. This structure helps keep the workshop focused and ensures that all participants leave with valuable, actionable knowledge. Clear goals also facilitate a more organized flow, allowing time for demonstrations, discussions, and hands-on activities. Securing a venue that supports interactive learning is essential for those looking to host a workshop. A local community center or library could provide the space for group activities and discussions.

The diversity of perspectives in workshops is one of their greatest strengths. When people from different age groups and backgrounds come together, the exchange of ideas becomes rich and multifaceted. Each participant brings their own experiences and insights, contributing to a collective pool of knowledge. This variety fosters open dialogue and idea exchange, encouraging participants to consider different viewpoints and strategies. For instance, a younger participant might introduce a new digital tool for tracking DMSO usage, while a senior member might share wisdom gained from years of personal experience. These interactions not only enrich the learning process but also build a sense of community and mutual respect among participants.

Past workshops have shown just how impactful this collaborative learning can be. Consider one case where a workshop led to a breakthrough in DMSO use. Participants, guided by an expert, experimented with different DMSO concentrations, leading to the discovery of an optimal formula for treating a specific condition. This collective effort not only benefited those present but also contributed to the broader community's understanding of DMSO applications. Another testimonial from a workshop attendee highlights the friendships formed through shared learning experiences. This individual found a sense of belonging and ongoing support from peers who understood their health challenges, illustrating these gatherings' lasting impact. These workshops become more than just educational sessions; they evolve into supportive networks where learning and growth are continuous, driven by the collective energy and enthusiasm of the group.

## BUILDING A SUPPORT SYSTEM: FAMILY AND FRIENDS INVOLVEMENT

Navigating health changes or exploring new treatments like DMSO is rarely a solitary endeavor. Involving family and friends can make a significant difference, offering a foundation of emotional encouragement and practical support. The people closest to you provide not only motivation but also a reassuring presence that can boost your confidence as you try something new. They can be instrumental in reminding you of your progress, celebrating small victories, and offering comfort during setbacks. The journey to improved health often involves ups and downs, and having loved ones by your side can make these fluctuations more manageable.

Family and friends can also assist with the practical aspects of DMSO application and monitoring. Having a trusted person to help you apply DMSO, especially in hard-to-reach areas, can ensure that you adhere to the recommended protocols. This assistance can prevent overuse or misapplication, which might lead to skin irritation. Additionally, they can help track any changes in symptoms or side effects, providing an extra layer of observation that can be invaluable. This partnership turns health management into a collaborative effort, reducing the feeling of isolation that can sometimes accompany chronic conditions.

Effective communication is key to involving loved ones in your DMSO use. Start by educating them about its benefits and safety. Share your research and information, helping them understand why you chose this path. Address any concerns they might have openly and encourage them to ask questions. This dialogue fosters trust and understanding, ensuring that they feel comfortable and informed. It also empowers them to support you better as they gain insight into your treatment plan and its potential impact.

Consider organizing family meetings or casual gatherings to discuss your health goals and how DMSO fits into them. These sessions provide a platform to share updates, discuss challenges, and explore solutions together. Encouraging loved ones to participate in this process strengthens your support network and enhances the sense of unity and shared purpose. It transforms health management into a collective endeavor where each person plays a role in fostering wellness.

Collaborative approaches to wellness extend beyond discussions. Engaging in family wellness activities can amplify the benefits of DMSO. Activities like group walks, yoga sessions, or cooking healthy meals together promote a holistic approach to health that complements your treatment. These activities also provide opportunities for bonding, reinforcing the emotional connections that underpin your support system. Sharing resources, such as articles or books on DMSO and related health topics, further enriches this collaborative approach. It creates a shared knowledge base that empowers everyone involved, enhancing the overall effectiveness of your wellness plan.

Real-life stories highlight the transformative power of involving family and friends. Consider the story of a family member assisting with the DMSO application to improve mobility. Their consistent support ensured proper application and moral support that boosted the individual's confidence. This collaboration resulted in improved mobility and a strengthened bond between them. Another testimonial involves friends sharing tips and encouragement in a local group. Their collective experiences and insights offered practical advice and emotional support, helping each member navigate their health journey more easily.

Involving loved ones in your health endeavors enriches the experience, turning it into a shared journey of discovery and growth. Their support provides a safety net, fostering resilience and optimism as you explore new treatment options. This chapter has explored the invaluable role that family and friends play in enhancing your DMSO experience, emphasizing the need for open communication and collaboration. As you progress, remember that these connections are supportive and integral to achieving your health goals. Together, you can navigate the complexities of health and wellness, finding strength in unity and shared purpose.

9

# ENHANCING OVERALL WELLNESS WITH DMSO

Imagine waking up each day with a sense of anticipation, knowing you have tools to support your well-being. For many, establishing a routine is the cornerstone of maintaining health and stability, and integrating DMSO into this routine can offer profound benefits. The power of a routine lies in its ability to transform daily habits into meaningful practices that contribute to both physical and mental well-being. Just like brushing your teeth or taking a brisk morning walk, the regular application of DMSO can become a steadfast element of your health regimen, offering stability and predictability in a chaotic world.

Routine plays a pivotal role in maximizing the benefits of DMSO, helping to ensure consistent and effective use. Incorporating DMSO into your morning and evening rituals becomes a natural part of your day, seamlessly woven into your existing habits. This consistency is key to achieving long-term benefits. Over time, regular use can help reduce inflammation, alleviate pain, and even improve skin health. By establishing a routine, you eliminate the guesswork and make the DMSO application a non-negotiable part of your self-care, enhancing its effectiveness and ensuring you reap its full benefits.

To seamlessly integrate DMSO into your daily life, consider pairing its application with other self-care activities. For instance, you might apply DMSO during your morning quiet time as you sip a cup of herbal tea or engage in a few moments of meditation. In the evening, it can be part of your wind-down routine, following a warm bath or gentle stretching exercises. Using reminders or habit trackers can also be incredibly helpful. These tools can prompt you to apply DMSO simultaneously each day, reinforcing the habit until it becomes second nature. This structured approach not only ensures consistency but also reduces decision fatigue, freeing up mental space for other pursuits.

The impact of a well-established routine extends beyond the physical. It also fosters mental clarity and focus. When you know exactly what to expect from your day, you can approach life's challenges clearly. This predictability can reduce stress and anxiety, creating a calm and centered mindset. For many, the act of caring for oneself—of dedicating time and attention to personal health—promotes a sense of empowerment and control. This mental shift can be just as transformative as the physical benefits of DMSO, supporting a holistic sense of wellness that encompasses both body and mind.

Consider the story of Linda, a dedicated gardener who found new joy in her hobby through consistent DMSO use. By applying DMSO each morning before heading out to her garden, Linda noticed a marked improvement in her joint flexibility, allowing her to spend more time tending to her beloved plants. Similarly, Sam, a retired teacher, found relief from the persistent discomfort of arthritis through a simple evening routine. By incorporating the DMSO application into his nightly ritual of reading and reflection,

Sam experienced enhanced mobility and reduced pain, enabling him to resume his cherished walks in the park.

**Reflection Section: Your Ideal Routine**

Take a moment to reflect on your daily routine. How might DMSO fit into your morning or evening rituals? Consider the activities that bring joy and peace and how DMSO can complement these moments. Jot down your thoughts and create a plan for integrating DMSO into your life, focusing on consistency and enjoyment.

These stories highlight the transformative power of routine. By making DMSO a regular part of their lives, Linda and Sam not only improved their physical well-being but also enhanced their overall quality of life. Their experiences serve as an inspiring reminder that small, consistent actions can lead to significant changes. As you consider incorporating DMSO into your routine, remember that the journey to wellness is deeply personal. Embrace the process and celebrate each step forward, knowing that your commitment to a routine will support your health and vitality in the days and years to come.

## MIND-BODY CONNECTION: STRESS MANAGEMENT WITH DMSO

Stress is an omnipresent force that affects our health in profound ways, often creeping into our lives unnoticed. Physically, it manifests as tension, headaches, and fatigue, while mentally, it can cloud our thoughts and sap our joy. Understanding the physiological effects of stress is crucial; it triggers the release of hormones like cortisol, which in excess can lead to inflammation, disrupt sleep, and weaken the immune system. Over time, this can erode our well-being, leaving us vulnerable to various ailments. DMSO, known for its versatility, offers a unique way to support the nervous system and help manage stress. When applied topically, it can relax tense muscles and ease discomfort, providing a soothing balm to the physical manifestations of stress. By working on a cellular level, DMSO may help to calm the signals that exacerbate anxiety and tension, offering a respite from the relentless pressure that stress can impose.

Incorporating DMSO into stress management routines can be both practical and effective. Applying it to areas where tension accumulates, such as the neck, shoulders, or back, can provide immediate relief from physical discomfort. This is particularly beneficial during stressful times when muscles tend to tighten and ache. Integrating DMSO application into relaxation rituals like meditation can enhance the calming effects, creating a more profound sense of peace. Imagine sitting in a quiet room, with soft music playing, as you gently massage DMSO into your temples or shoulders. The aroma, while distinctive, becomes part of a comforting routine, grounding you in the present moment and helping to dissolve the day's worries.

Pairing DMSO with complementary stress-reduction practices magnifies its benefits. Breathing exercises, for instance, are a simple yet powerful way to harness the mind-body connection. By focusing on slow, deep breaths, you signal your body to relax, lowering heart rate and blood pressure, which DMSO can complement by easing physical tension. Mindfulness practices, such as guided imagery, can also be enhanced with DMSO. As you visualize serene landscapes or calming scenes, the application of DMSO can serve as a tactile anchor, drawing your attention away from stressors and into a space of tranquility. Herbal teas, like chamomile or lavender, and aromatherapy can further enhance relaxation, creating a multi-sensory experience that soothes both mind and body.

Real-life stories highlight DMSO's role in stress management, offering hope and inspiration. Consider the experience of James, a retired engineer who faced high-pressure situations throughout his career. After discovering DMSO, he began applying it to his neck and shoulders during stressful meetings. This ritual became a source of calm, allowing him to approach challenges with a clearer mind and steadier hand. Another voice is that of Anne, a busy grandmother who juggled family responsibilities and volunteer work. She found that incorporating DMSO into her evening routine, alongside a cup of herbal tea and quiet reflection, significantly reduced her anxiety levels. The physical relaxation she experienced opened the door to deeper mental calm, transforming her evenings into a time of rejuvenation rather than stress.

These stories underscore the potential of DMSO as a tool for managing stress, offering both physical relief and a pathway to mental clarity. By understanding how stress affects us and exploring how DMSO can counteract these effects, you can find new avenues for calm and balance in your life. The simple act of caring for your body with DMSO can become a ritual of self-compassion, helping you navigate life's challenges with greater ease. The key lies in embracing this practice as part of a broader strategy, one that honors both the body and mind in the pursuit of well-being.

## LONG-TERM HEALTH GOALS: USING DMSO FOR LONGEVITY

The concept of longevity extends beyond simply adding years to life; it embodies the vitality and quality of those years. As we age, the focus shifts towards preventative care and maintaining wellness to ensure that we live longer and well. This shift is crucial, particularly for aging individuals who desire to fully preserve their independence and enjoy life. Prioritizing long-term health means embracing strategies that support your body's natural processes and mitigate age-related decline. In this context, DMSO emerges as a valuable ally, offering benefits that extend beyond immediate relief to support sustained health and vitality.

DMSO's potential in promoting longevity lies in its ability to support cellular health and regeneration. At a cellular level, DMSO enhances the body's natural repair mechanisms, helping maintain the integrity and function of cells as they age. This not only bolsters cellular resilience but also aids in the regeneration of tissues, which is vital for maintaining overall health. Additionally, DMSO's anti-inflammatory properties play a significant role in reducing age-related decline. Chronic inflammation is a known contributor to various age-related diseases, and by mitigating inflammation, DMSO helps protect against conditions that can erode quality of life over time. This dual action—supporting cell repair and reducing inflammation—positions DMSO as a promising component of a longevity-focused health plan.

Setting and achieving long-term health goals with DMSO requires a thoughtful approach. Start by identifying your personal health priorities. Consider what aspects of health are most important to you, whether it's maintaining mobility, supporting cognitive function, or enhancing skin health. Once these priorities are clear, you can set realistic and attainable objectives aligning with your overall health vision. Tracking your progress is essential in this process. Regularly assess how DMSO impacts your health, and be open to adjusting your goals as needed. This flexibility allows you to respond to changes in your health and ensures that your approach remains effective and aligned with your evolving needs.

The experiences of those who have integrated DMSO into their long-term health plans offer valuable insights. Take, for instance, the story of Robert, a retired architect who prioritized maintaining his energy levels and vitality. By incorporating DMSO into his regimen, Robert found that he could sustain his active lifestyle, participating in activities he loved, like hiking and gardening. DMSO's consistent support to his joints and muscles was instrumental in preserving his independence. Another inspiring example is Margaret, who focused on sustaining her joint health. With the help of DMSO, she managed to keep her arthritis symptoms at bay, ensuring that she could continue enjoying daily walks and social engagements without discomfort. These stories highlight the transformative power of DMSO in supporting long-term health goals, demonstrating its potential to enhance longevity and the quality of life accompanying it.

As you consider your long-term health goals, consider how DMSO can fit into the broader picture of your wellness strategy. By focusing on preventative care and embracing DMSO's unique properties, you can extend your lifespan and enrich it with vitality and joy. Prioritizing longevity is not just about adding years to life but about ensuring those years are filled with health, happiness, and fulfillment.

## HOLISTIC HEALTH: EMBRACING A BALANCED LIFESTYLE

Holistic health is an approach that considers the whole person—mind, body, and spirit—in the pursuit of wellness. It is about finding balance and harmony in every aspect of life. Rather than solely treating symptoms, holistic health emphasizes prevention and natural healing. It encourages you to listen to your body and mind, recognizing the interconnectedness of all your systems. This approach values the integration of various wellness practices to promote overall health. By nurturing the mind, body, and spirit, you create a foundation for sustained well-being. This balanced perspective is essential in a world that prioritizes quick fixes over lasting solutions.

DMSO plays a significant role in a holistic health strategy. Its ability to support detoxification and overall cellular health makes it a valuable component of any wellness plan. DMSO complements other wellness practices beautifully by aiding in removing toxins and supporting the body's natural repair processes. DMSO can enhance these efforts by following a balanced diet, exercising regularly, or practicing mindfulness. It works in tandem with a healthy lifestyle, amplifying the benefits of your other wellness activities. This synergy helps you achieve a more profound sense of health and vitality, reinforcing the principles of holistic living.

To achieve a balanced lifestyle, creating a personalized wellness plan is crucial. Start by assessing your current habits and identifying areas for improvement. What aspects of your health need more attention? With this awareness, set realistic goals that align with your values and priorities. Incorporate practices that promote balance, such as regular physical activity, nutritious eating, and adequate rest. Mindfulness and gratitude are powerful tools for maintaining mental health. Taking a few moments each day to reflect on what you're thankful for can shift your mindset and promote emotional well-being. These small practices, integrated into daily life, contribute to a holistic approach to health.

The stories of individuals who have embraced a balanced lifestyle with DMSO are genuinely inspiring. Consider Sarah, who struggled with chronic fatigue and stress. By integrating DMSO into her wellness plan, she experienced an improvement in her energy levels and overall well-being. She found that using DMSO in conjunction with a plant-based diet and daily meditation helped her manage stress more effectively. This holistic approach not only improved her physical health but also enhanced her mental clarity and emotional resilience. Sarah's experience illustrates the potential of combining DMSO with other natural remedies to achieve a balanced, fulfilling life.

Another testament to the power of holistic health is John's story. After years of dealing with joint pain, John decided to take a more comprehensive approach. He began applying DMSO while making lifestyle changes that focused on whole foods and regular yoga practice. The combined effect was remarkable. His joint pain decreased, and he also found a renewed sense of balance and joy in everyday activities. For John, DMSO was a catalyst that supported his journey toward holistic health, helping him embrace life with renewed vigor.

These stories highlight the transformative potential of DMSO within a holistic framework. By embracing a balanced lifestyle, you can unlock new levels of health and happiness. Integrating mind, body, and spirit creates a ripple effect, positively impacting all aspects of your life. As you continue to explore the possibilities of DMSO, remember that true wellness is a journey, not a destination. Each step you take towards balance brings you closer to a healthier, more fulfilling life.

# 10

# THE FUTURE OF DMSO AND EMERGING THERAPIES

Picture a world where the smallest of innovations can have the biggest impact on health. That's the promise of the latest research in DMSO. Scientists are unveiling breakthroughs that could change how we use DMSO, making it more effective than ever. Imagine advanced delivery systems that allow DMSO to work faster and more efficiently. These new methods could revolutionize its use, providing relief with precision that was once thought impossible. Novel formulations now target specific needs, tailoring DMSO's application to individual conditions and maximizing its benefits. It's a step forward in personalizing care, ensuring that each use of DMSO is as effective as possible.

One of the most exciting developments is the use of nanotechnology. This field opens new horizons for DMSO, improving how the body absorbs it. Nanotechnology involves manipulating materials on an atomic or molecular scale, enhancing the bioavailability of substances. For DMSO, this means more efficient absorption, allowing it to reach areas previously inaccessible. The implications are vast, offering hope for conditions that require targeted treatment. Alongside nanotechnology, artificial intelligence also plays a role. AI-driven research is uncovering new applications for DMSO, analyzing vast amounts of data to predict outcomes and optimize its use. This technology-driven approach is setting the stage for smarter, more effective therapies.

Collaboration is another key to unlocking DMSO's potential. Universities, biotech companies, and researchers are joining forces to push the boundaries of what we know. These partnerships foster innovation, combining diverse expertise to explore DMSO's capabilities. Global initiatives are also in play, encouraging sharing research findings across borders. This collective effort accelerates discovery, ensuring that breakthroughs are not confined to one laboratory or country. By pooling resources and knowledge, the global community is paving the way for DMSO's next chapter, one characterized by innovation and collaboration.

The possibilities for DMSO extend into uncharted territories. Consider its potential in neuroprotective applications, where it could play a role in managing cognitive disorders. The ability of DMSO to penetrate deeply and deliver therapeutic agents makes it an intriguing candidate for addressing neurological issues. Imagine a future where DMSO supports brain health, offering new hope for conditions like Alzheimer's or Parkinson's. Beyond the brain, DMSO's role in regenerative medicine is gaining attention. Tissue engineering, a field focused on repairing or replacing damaged tissues, stands to benefit from DMSO's unique properties. In this context, DMSO could aid in developing new tissues, enhancing the body's natural healing processes.

These advancements are just the beginning. As research continues, the future of DMSO looks promising, marked by innovation and potential. It's a future where technology and collaboration drive discovery, expanding the horizons of what DMSO can achieve.

For those of us exploring natural remedies, these developments offer exciting opportunities. They represent a chance to tap into DMSO's full potential, leveraging the latest science to improve health and well-being. As we look ahead, the promise of DMSO continues to unfold, inviting us to explore its capabilities in ways we never thought possible. This journey is one of discovery, filled with new insights and possibilities that are waiting to be realized.

## DMSO AND EMERGING THERAPIES: WHAT'S NEXT?

DMSO is at the forefront of emerging therapies, offering a promising adjunct in integrative oncology. As cancer treatment evolves, there's a growing emphasis on combining conventional approaches with supportive therapies that enhance efficacy and reduce side effects. DMSO, with its ability to penetrate tissues and enhance the delivery of chemotherapy drugs, presents a unique opportunity in this field. It acts as a facilitator, potentially improving the efficacy of cancer treatments by ensuring that therapeutic agents reach their target tissues more effectively. This approach could reduce the dosage required, minimizing the adverse effects often associated with cancer therapies. By supporting the body's natural defenses while bolstering conventional treatments, DMSO is carving out a niche in the complex landscape of cancer care.

The integration of DMSO into advanced wound care technologies represents another exciting development. Wound healing is a complex process that can be hindered by factors such as infection and inflammation. DMSO, known for its anti-inflammatory and antimicrobial properties, is used in new formulations promoting faster and more effective healing. These technologies incorporate DMSO into wound dressings and topical treatments, enhancing tissue regeneration and reducing healing time. The potential to improve outcomes for patients with chronic wounds or those recovering from surgery is significant, offering a new layer of care that complements existing treatment protocols. This innovation not only addresses the physical aspects of wound healing but also the emotional toll that slow recovery can take on patients, providing a holistic approach to recovery.

Personalized medicine is another area where DMSO's potential is being realized. Tailoring treatments based on individual genetic and metabolic profiles is gaining traction. DMSO's role in this is multifaceted, offering a medium through which treatments can be customized to the individual's unique biological makeup. By considering factors such as genetic predispositions and metabolic responses, healthcare providers can develop patient-specific treatment plans that optimize outcomes. This level of customization ensures that therapies are not only more effective but also safer, minimizing the risk of adverse reactions. The integration of DMSO into these personalized plans highlights its versatility and adaptability, making it a valuable tool in the push toward more individualized healthcare solutions.

Regulatory developments are also shaping the future of DMSO use. As its applications expand, so do the guidelines governing its use. The FDA and international bodies continually update standards to reflect new research and clinical findings. These changes impact how DMSO is used and approved, influencing everything from labeling requirements to permissible concentrations in consumer products. New clinical trials are instrumental in this process, providing evidence to support regulatory approvals and expand DMSO's therapeutic reach. As these regulations evolve, they ensure that the use of DMSO remains safe and effective, balancing innovation with the need for oversight and control.

Emerging therapies utilizing DMSO are diverse and innovative. In stem cell therapy, DMSO is used as a cryoprotectant, preserving the viability and functionality of cells destined for transplantation. This application is crucial in regenerative medicine, where maintaining cell integrity is paramount. Additionally, DMSO's synergy with peptide-based therapies is being explored. Peptides, which are short chains of amino acids, have various therapeutic applications, from anti-aging treatments to hormone regulation. DMSO can enhance their delivery, ensuring that they reach the targeted tissues efficiently. These examples underscore the breadth of DMSO's applicability, highlighting how it can augment emerging treatments across different medical fields. As we continue to explore these therapies, DMSO's role in modern medicine becomes increasingly apparent, offering new avenues for health and healing that align with the evolving needs of patients and practitioners alike.

## EXPLORING NICOTINE: A HIDDEN BOMBSHELL FOR FOCUS AND ENERGY

Nicotine, often associated with tobacco and its adverse effects, emerges in a new light when considered for its cognitive benefits. This pivot in perception is intriguing, especially when you explore nicotine's role in enhancing focus and energy. There's a growing body of research suggesting nicotine's potential to sharpen cognitive function. It acts on the brain by influencing neurotransmitter activity, specifically the nicotinic acetylcholine receptors. These receptors play a crucial role in attention, learning, and memory. What if nicotine could be used to boost these cognitive domains, providing mental clarity without the harmful effects of smoking? It's a question that piques interest, especially for those looking for natural ways to enhance mental acuity.

The scientific basis for nicotine's effects is robust, supported by studies that delve into its impact on brain function. Research has shown that nicotine can improve short-term working memory and attention span. It acts as a mild stimulant, enhancing the release of neurotransmitters like dopamine and norepinephrine, which are pivotal for alertness and mood regulation. Long-term studies indicate potential neuroprotective benefits, hinting at its role in reducing the risk of neurodegenerative diseases like Alzheimer's. These findings position nicotine not just as a substance with addictive potential but as a compound with nuanced effects that could be harnessed for cognitive enhancement. Such insights challenge the traditional narrative, inviting a reconsideration of nicotine's place in wellness strategies.

The synergy between DMSO and nicotine presents a fascinating avenue for exploration. DMSO, known for enhancing other compounds' absorption, could amplify nicotine's effects. This combination raises possibilities for focus-driven therapies, where precise delivery and controlled use of nicotine could improve cognitive performance. Imagine a scenario where a small, controlled dose of nicotine, delivered efficiently through DMSO, offers a boost in focus and mental clarity. This application could extend to therapeutic settings, supporting individuals with cognitive deficits or those needing heightened concentration. While speculative, the potential for such synergy invites further investigation, offering a new dimension to both substances' applications. My next book will reveal the answers and research.

*Interactive Element: Reflection Section*

Consider your perspective on nicotine's role in wellness. Reflect on the following prompts:

- How do you view nicotine's potential as a cognitive enhancer?
- What concerns or questions arise when considering its use alongside DMSO?
- How might ethical considerations shape your opinion on using nicotine in health strategies if it were proven NOT addictive?

Document your reflections and revisit them as you explore this topic further. This exercise encourages critical thinking and helps clarify your stance on this complex issue.

## DMSO IN THE NEXT DECADE: PREDICTIONS AND POSSIBILITIES

In the coming decade, DMSO stands poised to make its mark firmly within mainstream medicine. As researchers and practitioners continue to uncover its multifaceted benefits, its integration into more conventional treatments seems inevitable. We may witness DMSO being prescribed more frequently alongside standard medications, particularly in areas like pain management, where it offers a natural alternative with fewer side effects. This shift could redefine how both doctors and patients view natural therapies, positioning DMSO as a bridge between holistic and medical approaches. It's an exciting prospect, considering how its unique properties can complement existing treatments, potentially enhancing their effectiveness and patient outcomes.

Beyond the medical field, DMSO's applications could also expand into non-medical areas. Industries such as skincare and wellness will likely explore DMSO's potential for enhancing product efficacy. Imagine skincare lines that leverage DMSO's ability to improve the penetration of active ingredients, offering deeper hydration and rejuvenation without the need for invasive procedures. The wellness sector, always looking for natural enhancements, might incorporate DMSO into relaxation therapies or sports recovery products, capitalizing on its soothing and anti-inflammatory properties. These explorations could lead to innovative products that appeal to consumers seeking natural solutions for everyday health and beauty challenges.

Yet, as with any promising development, challenges accompany opportunities. One primary hurdle will be addressing safety concerns and public perception. Despite its benefits, DMSO's past controversies linger in public consciousness. Educating the public about its safety and proper use will be crucial. This involves transparent communication from manufacturers and healthcare providers about its benefits and potential side effects. Additionally, with the growing interest in natural therapies, there's an opportunity to position DMSO as a safe, effective choice within this trend. As more people turn to natural remedies, DMSO could find its place as a trusted component of a holistic health regimen, provided its presentation is honest and informed.

Global health trends will also influence DMSO's trajectory. As populations age, the demand for solutions that address aging-related issues, such as joint pain and cognitive decline, will soar. DMSO's potential anti-aging and cognitive support applications align perfectly with these needs, offering a natural option that fits the larger wellness culture. People are becoming more proactive about their health, seeking ways to maintain vitality as they age. DMSO could meet this demand, becoming a staple in pursuing longevity and quality of life. Its versatility and ease of use make it an attractive option for those looking to support their health naturally.

Innovation will play a pivotal role in shaping DMSO's future. Advances in biotechnology could lead to improved formulations that enhance its effectiveness and reduce any side effects. These breakthroughs might involve refining how DMSO interacts with other compounds, ensuring optimal delivery and uptake within the body. Digital health tools could also revolutionize how DMSO is used. Imagine apps that track your health metrics, offering personalized recommendations for DMSO use based on your unique needs. These tools could provide data-driven insights, helping you make informed decisions about your health routine. Such innovations promise to make DMSO not only more accessible but also more precisely tailored to individual needs.

As these changes unfold, DMSO's role in health and wellness is set to grow, offering new possibilities for enhancing well-being. The next decade could see it becoming a fixture in both medical and everyday health practices, supported by a foundation of scientific research and technological advancement.

## PREPARING FOR THE FUTURE: STAYING INFORMED AND ENGAGED

In a world constantly evolving with new health discoveries, staying informed about DMSO developments is more crucial than ever. Subscribing to scientific journals and newsletters can be an excellent way to keep up-to-date. These resources provide the latest findings, studies, and expert opinions on DMSO's applications and potential. By reading these publications, you gain insights into ongoing research, which can help you understand new uses and safety protocols. Journals such as *The Journal of*

*Alternative and Complementary Medicine* often feature peer-reviewed articles that delve into the nuances of DMSO, offering reliable information that can guide your decisions.

Engaging actively with the DMSO community can also enhance your understanding and application of this compound. Joining professional organizations or attending conferences allows you to network with researchers and practitioners who share your interest in natural remedies. These events provide a platform for exchanging ideas, discussing challenges, and learning from others' experiences. Conferences often feature workshops and presentations that can deepen your knowledge and introduce you to cutting-edge techniques. This engagement fosters a sense of community, where you can find support and inspiration from like-minded individuals pursuing similar health goals.

Participating in online forums and discussion groups is another way to stay connected and informed. These platforms enable you to ask questions, share experiences, and receive feedback from diverse users. The collective wisdom found in these communities can be invaluable, offering practical tips and firsthand accounts of DMSO use. Whether discussing dosage adjustments, application methods, or potential side effects, these groups provide open dialogue and learning space. By contributing to these conversations, you also build a supportive community that values shared knowledge and growth.

While exploring new information, it's vital to maintain a level of critical thinking and skepticism. Not all sources are created equal, and assessing the credibility of information is key. Look for studies backed by reputable institutions and consider the authors' qualifications. Balancing optimism with scientific rigor ensures that you're making informed decisions based on facts rather than hype. By questioning and verifying the information you

# THE FUTURE OF DMSO AND EMERGING THERAPIES | 119

encounter, you can discern which developments are groundbreaking and which might be overstated. This approach safeguards against misinformation, ensuring that your choices are grounded in reliable evidence.

For continued learning and exploration, a variety of resources are available. Books focused on advanced DMSO topics can provide comprehensive insights and detailed guidance. Titles such as *DMSO: Nature's Healer* offer in-depth analysis and practical advice for integrating DMSO into your health regimen. Online courses and webinars are also valuable tools, offering structured learning experiences that delve into specific aspects of DMSO use. These courses often feature expert instructors who can answer questions and provide personalized feedback. By seeking out these resources, you equip yourself with the knowledge needed to navigate the ever-evolving landscape of DMSO and its applications.

As we explore the potential of DMSO, staying informed and engaged becomes an ongoing process of learning and adaptation. With each discovery, you have the opportunity to refine your approach, ensuring that your use of DMSO remains effective and safe. By actively participating in the community, subscribing to reliable sources, and maintaining a critical eye, you position yourself at the forefront of this exciting field. Embrace the possibilities that come with this knowledge, and continue to explore the vast potential that DMSO holds for enhancing your health and well-being.

# CONCLUSION

As we reach the end of this book, I invite you to reflect on the transformative journey we've embarked upon together. We started with a simple curiosity about DMSO, a compound that might have seemed mysterious or even controversial to some. Through personal stories and extensive research, we've explored its potential as a natural healer, uncovering how it can profoundly impact health and well-being. My journey with DMSO began out of necessity; after years of battling chronic pain and health issues, I discovered a path to relief and vitality that I could not keep to myself. It is this journey that I have shared with you, hoping to illuminate a pathway that offers hope and healing.

This book was born from a vision to empower you, especially if you are an adult or senior, with the knowledge needed to make informed health decisions. The world of natural healing can often feel overwhelming, filled with choices and claims that are difficult to navigate. I aimed to simplify this to provide you with clear, evidence-based insights into how DMSO can be a part of your wellness toolkit. By understanding its properties and applications, you can confidently explore its use as a viable option for managing pain, reducing inflammation, and boosting energy and vitality.

Throughout the book, we delve into key learnings that form the foundation of understanding DMSO. We examine its scientific basis, safe application techniques, and role in managing chronic conditions like arthritis and skin health. We also consider its place in a holistic lifestyle, complementing other natural remedies and wellness practices. Each chapter was crafted to provide you with a comprehensive view of DMSO's potential, grounded in both personal experience and scientific research.

As you consider the next steps in your health journey, I encourage you to take action. Explore DMSO as part of your wellness plan and consult healthcare professionals for personalized advice. Start small, perhaps with a single application, and observe how your body responds. Remember that DMSO is not a cure-all; it is a tool that, when used wisely, can support your body's natural healing processes. Be open to integrating it alongside other treatments and lifestyle changes that align with your health goals.

I also urge you to stay curious and engaged with ongoing developments in DMSO research. Science is ever-evolving, and discoveries can enhance our understanding and application of this remarkable compound. Engage with communities, whether online or locally, to share experiences and learn from others. These connections can provide support and encouragement, enriching your journey and expanding your knowledge.

Sharing your experiences can be immensely powerful. Consider writing testimonials, participating in forums, or joining local support groups. Doing so contributes to a growing community of individuals exploring natural healing options. Your story could inspire others, giving them the courage to try something new and transformative.

As I conclude, I want to express my heartfelt gratitude for your engagement with this book. Your willingness to explore DMSO and other natural remedies reflects your commitment to your health. I hope that the insights shared here will lead you to improved health and vitality, allowing you to live each day with greater freedom and joy.

The takeaway from this journey is one of empowerment. You now possess the knowledge and insights to make informed choices about DMSO and other natural healing options. Embrace this empowerment, and let it guide you as you continue to explore the possibilities. Here's to a future filled with health, vitality, and the wisdom to navigate your wellness journey with confidence.

# DMSO FOR ADULTS AND SENIORS
## YOUR GUIDE TO NATURAL HEALING

**Relieve Chronic Pain · Reduce Inflammation · Renew Energy**

*"The best way to find yourself is to lose yourself in the service of others."*

— MAHATMA GANDHI

When we help others, we not only brighten their lives but also bring more joy to our own. Together, we can make a difference!

Would you like to help someone—just like you—who's looking for relief from pain or wondering how to feel better every day?

My goal with *DMSO for Adults and Seniors* is to make it a helpful guide for anyone exploring the benefits of natural remedies.

But here's the thing: most people choose books based on reviews. That's where you come in!

Your review doesn't just help me—it helps someone else who's curious about DMSO but unsure where to start. By sharing your thoughts, you can make a big impact.

**Why Your Review Matters**

When you leave a review, you help:

- Someone find hope and relief from pain.
- A small business grow and give back to its community.
- An entrepreneur provide for their family.

- A reader take the first step toward a healthier, happier life.

It's easy, free, and takes just a minute, but your words could change someone's journey with DMSO forever.

**How to Leave Your Review**

1. Visit this link or scan the QR code below:
2. [https://www.amazon.com/review/review-your-purchases/?asin=BOOKASIN]
3. Share your honest thoughts. (Even one sentence is helpful!)

If you're the kind of person who loves helping others, then you're exactly who I wrote this book for. Thank you for supporting this mission and helping more people discover the power of DMSO.

With heartfelt thanks,

MT Vessel

# REFERENCES

*Dimethyl sulfoxide* https://en.wikipedia.org/wiki/Dimethyl_sulfoxide

*DMSO (Dimethyl Sulfoxide): Uses, Benefits, Risks, and More* https://www.healthline.com/health/what-is-dmso

*DMSO for Arthritis: Does It Help?* https://www.healthline.com/health/arthritis/dmso-for-arthritis

*Dimethyl sulfoxide* https://en.wikipedia.org/wiki/Dimethyl_sulfoxide

*Dimethyl Sulfoxide (DMSO)* https://hci-portal.hci.utah.edu/sites/factsheets/Shared%20Documents/dimethyl-sulfoxide-dmso.pdf?Mobile=1

*Dimethyl Sulfoxide Dosage Guide + Max Dose, Adjustments* https://www.drugs.com/dosage/dimethyl-sulfoxide.html

*Adverse reactions of dimethyl sulfoxide in humans* https://pmc.ncbi.nlm.nih.gov/articles/PMC6707402/

*LCSS: DIMETHYL SULFOXIDE* https://web.stanford.edu/dept/EHS/cgi-bin/lcst/lcss/lcss33.html

*DMSO Represses Inflammatory Cytokine Production From ...* https://pubmed.ncbi.nlm.nih.gov/27031833/

*Efficacy of a topical treatment protocol with dimethyl ...* https://pubmed.ncbi.nlm.nih.gov/22266201/

*Efficacy and safety of topical diclofenac containing dimethyl ...* https://www.sciencedirect.com/science/article/abs/pii/S0304395909001584

*The Untapped Healing Potential of DMSO* https://www.lifeextension.com/magazine/2007/7/cover_dmso?srsltid=AfmBOootAjAoUS35tM7vQQMgCe9bYxKLbuT5wN9pIr4_T3XiLR9fgqHI

*Dimethyl Sulfoxide: History, Chemistry, and Clinical Utility ...* https://pmc.ncbi.nlm.nih.gov/articles/PMC3460663/

*DMSO – Health Information Library* https://www.peacehealth.org/medical-topics/id/hn-2839006

*Low-concentration DMSO accelerates skin wound healing ...* https://pubmed.ncbi.nlm.nih.gov/32167156/

*1832-Hypersensitivity reaction to dimethyl sulfoxide (DMSO)* https://www.eviq.org.au/clinical-resources/side-effect-and-toxicity-management/immunological/1832-hypersensitivity-reaction-to-dimethyl-sulfoxi

*A Natural Alliance: Castor Oil and DMSO for Joint Pain Relief* https://barecatbody.

com/blogs/news/a-natural-alliance-castor-oil-and-dmso-for-joint-pain-relief?srsltid=AfmBOoogrHRImlkCnbIJdlVzr2BiMMZuH6Ja-XWwftcK78GGMbmOLm8

*10 Supplements That Fight Inflammation* https://www.healthline.com/nutrition/anti-inflammatory-supplements

*9 Benefits of Yoga | Johns Hopkins Medicine* https://www.hopkinsmedicine.org/health/wellness-and-prevention/9-benefits-of-yoga#:

*Alternative Therapies for Traditional Disease States* https://www.aafp.org/pubs/afp/issues/2003/0115/p339.html

*Dimethyl Sulfoxide: History, Chemistry, and Clinical Utility ...* https://pmc.ncbi.nlm.nih.gov/articles/PMC3460663/

*DMSO: Uses and Risks* https://www.webmd.com/vitamins-and-supplements/dmso-uses-and-risks

*Immunomodulatory effects and potential clinical ...* https://www.sciencedirect.com/science/article/pii/S0171298519303729

*Adverse reactions of dimethyl sulfoxide in humans* https://pmc.ncbi.nlm.nih.gov/articles/PMC6707402/

*Dimethyl Sulfoxide - DMSO Supplier and Distributor of Bulk ...* https://www.covalentchemical.com/chemical-distributor/dimethyl-sulfoxide--dmso-supplier-10218.aspx

*Dimethyl Sulfoxide (USP, BP, Ph. Eur.) pharma grade* https://www.itwreagents.com/rest-of-world/en/product/dimethyl-sulfoxide-usp-bp-ph-eur-pharma-grade/191954

*Cost effectiveness and cost utility of acetylcysteine versus ...* https://pubmed.ncbi.nlm.nih.gov/12515575/

*The Benefits of Combining DMSO and Essential Oils* https://herbalmana.com/blogs/herbal-mana-blog/the-benefits-of-combining-dmso-and-essential-oils

*Forum for Integrative Medicine* https://forumforintegrativemedicine.org/

*DMSO - Interstitial cystitis - Inspire* https://www.inspire.com/groups/interstitial-cystitis-association/discussion/dmso-kfq0cf/

*Hosting Community Health Workshops A Guide For Practices* https://nechayappraisals.com/hosting-community-health-workshops-a-guide-for-practices/

*Family Support and Well-being - ECLKC - HHS.gov* https://eclkc.ohs.acf.hhs.gov/family-support-well-being

*DMSO: Uses and Risks* https://www.webmd.com/vitamins-and-supplements/dmso-uses-and-risks

*DMSO + Castor Oil: All-Natural Remedy for Chronic Pain, ...* https://alivenhealthy.com/posts/dmso-castor-oil-all-natural-remedy-for-chronic-pain-inflammation-and-adhesions

*Holistic Approach to Fighting Inflammation* https://centrespringmd.com/holistic-approach-fighting-inflammation/?srsltid=AfmBOor9-V3mOiSqtQzyTlbCrKoA jAn97Y_wprVc60GePuTOzonj5evH

Cognitive Effects of Nicotine: Recent Progress - PMC https://pmc.ncbi.nlm.nih.gov/articles/PMC6018192/

DMSO induces drastic changes in human cellular ... https://www.nature.com/articles/s41598-019-40660-0

Application of nanotechnology in improving bioavailability ... https://pmc.ncbi.nlm.nih.gov/articles/PMC3959237/

Cognitive Effects of Nicotine: Recent Progress - PMC https://pmc.ncbi.nlm.nih.gov/articles/PMC6018192/#:

DMSO, cryopreservation & regenerative medicine https://www.regmednet.com/dimethyl-sulfoxide-alternatives-and-improvements-for-regenerative-medicine/

Benefits, Methods, and Practical Tips - Machine RFQ. https://www.machinerfq.com/abs-acetone-smoothing.html

Muscle Intelligence. https://muscleintelligence.libsyn.com/website/2022/12

Cream-soap-scrub for face with berry extract — 150 ml — Nuard Cosmetics | MakeUpHye. https://makeuphye.com/en/p/nuard-cosmetics/cream-soap-scrub-for-face-with-berry-extract/150-ml

Look Younger with This Anti-Aging Plant. https://www.institutefornaturalhealing.com/2012/12/look-younger-with-this-anti-aging-plant/

Marine Collagen - QIYOI Cosmética natural antiarrugas. https://qiyoi.com/en/natural-ingredients/marine-collagen/

Multifaceted Benefits of Lemon Oil for Skin: From Daily Care to Natural Deodorising. https://natrlskincare.co.uk/blogs/news/multifaceted-benefits-of-lemon-oil-for-skin-from-daily-care-to-natural-deodorising

Lewicka, K., Szymanek, I., Rogacz, D., Wrzalik, M., Łagiewka, J., Nowik-Zając, A., Zawierucha, I., Coseri, S., Puiu, I., Falfushynska, H., Rychter, P., & Rychter, P. (2024). Current Trends of Polymer Materials' Application in Agriculture. Sustainability, 16(19), 8439.

First Ever FDA-Approved Autonomous AI Diagnostic System | Evolving Science. https://www.evolving-science.com/intelligent-machines/ai-diagnostic-system-00776

Breathing Easy: Traditional Chinese Medicine Perspectives on COPD Management - Blog. https://heshoutang.com/naturo-library/diseases-in-naturo/breathing-easy-traditional-chinese-medicine-perspectives-on-copd-management

Disinfestation - Pest Control Cyprus | Nicosia. https://expresspestcy.com/disinfestation-2/?lang=en

What Is Hybrid Infrastructure? - Evocative Data Centers. https://evocative.com/resources/glossary/what-is-hybrid-infrastructure/

Cracking the Code: How to Read Food Labels for Hidden Sugars – Ditch The Guilt. https://ditchtheguilt.fit/blogs/news/cracking-the-code-how-to-read-food-labels-for-hidden-sugars

HOI CBD Broad Spectrum – House of Imhotep. https://houseofimhotep.com/products/hoi-cbd

Betty Kamen - Empowering Your Health with Wisdom and Wellness – Inspired by Dr. Betty Kamen. http://www.bettykamen.com/

Purchase and today price of baby powder talc - Bariteh. https://mineralsbuy.com/purchase-and-today-price-of-baby-powder-talc/

EMS Or TENS For Tendonitis - iTENS Australia. https://itens.com.au/ems-or-tens-for-tendonitis/

Revealing the UAE's Corporate Tax Landscape: What You Need to Know - AMD Audit. https://www.amdaudit.com/revealing-the-uaes-corporate-tax-landscape-what-you-need-to-know/

Natural alternative to metoprolol. https://metoprolol24h.top/natural-alternative-to-metoprolol/

Buy Propecia No Prescription. http://opkorenal.com/news/html/propecia.html

Crafting A Healthy Canine: Unveiling The Secrets Of An Effective Dog Diet Plan. https://psxcosmicvalues.com/crafting-a-healthy-canine-unveiling-the-secrets-of-an-effective-dog-diet-plan/

KOTC: X-Treme Fusion Gummies 800mg. https://wowrochester.com/edibles/kotc-fusion-gummies-800mg/

Medical Marijuana for Arthritis: Understanding the Benefits of CBD and THC on Pain, Inflammation, and Quality of Life. https://www.arcannabisclinic.com/how-marijuana-helps-with-severe-arthritis

Are Personal Injury Settlements Taxable in Florida? - Morgan Law Group, P.A.. https://policyadvocate.com/blog/are-personal-injury-settlements-taxable-in-florida/

Anti-Inflammatory Write For Us - Guest Post, Contribute, and Submit Post. https://www.healthremodeling.com/anti-inflammatory-write-for-us/

VARIOUS BENEFITS OF OSTEOPATHY SERVICE FOR HEALTH - ifvod.io. https://ifvod.io/various-benefits-of-osteopathy-service-for-health/

5 At-Home Remedies That Can Help Ease Your Sciatica Discomfort. https://backpainclinicbelleville.com/2024/01/02/5-at-home-remedies-that-can-help-ease-your-sciatica-discomfort/

The Importance of Strength Training After 55: Transform Your Health and Life. https://www.getgritstrong.com/blog-post/the-importance-of-strength-training-after-55-transform-your-health-and-life

St. Albans Group Health Insurance & Employee Benefit Plans. https://www.taylorbenefitsinsurance.com/st-albans-group-health-insurance-employee-benefit-plans/

Peroneal Tendon Pain Alternative Treatments | ReCELLebrate. https://recellebrate.com/stem-cell/treatments-for-peroneal-tendon-pain/

When To Call A Professional For Shower Plumbing. https://www.hawthorneplumberpros.com/emergency-plumber/when-to-call-a-professional-for-shower-plumbing/

Alternative for metoprolol. https://metoprolol24h.top/alternative-for-metoprolol/

Topical CBD products: what are they and how do they work? - HempWell CBD. https://hempwell.co.uk/topical-cbd-products-what-are-they-and-how-do-they-work/

Beyond Opioids: Harnessing the Power of Medicinal Marijuana for Chronic Pain Relief - Busk Wales. https://buskwales.co.uk/health-fitness/beyond-opioids-harnessing-the-power-of-medicinal-marijuana-for-chronic-pain-relief/

Local vs. International: Which Cabinet Supplier is Best for You? - New Design Concepts. https://thendcway.com/blog/2024/07/local-vs-international-which-cabinet-supplier-is-best-for-you/

Boost hydration with T-Sonic Technology | FOREO-Live Back Office. https://www.foreo.com/mysa/boost-hydration-with-t-sonic-technology/

Can growing pollution cause skin problems? - Intreviews. https://intreviews.com/can-growing-pollution-cause-skin-problems/

Unlocking the Healing Potential: Hyperbaric Oxygen Therapy for Wounds. https://www.thewoundpros.com/post/unlocking-the-healing-potential-hyperbaric-oxygen-therapy-for-wounds

Best Pure Shilajit to Use. https://grassit.co/blogs/a-comprehensive-guide-to-the-uses-and-benefits-of-purely-natural-shilajit/a-comprehensive-guide-to-the-uses-and-benefits-of-purely-natural-shilajit

Can You Mix Ferulic Acid With Retinol? | Ferulic Acid Serum. https://www.ferulicacidserum.com/blog/can-you-mix-ferulic-acid-with-retinol

Do You Have to Use a CPAP Machine Forever? • Surviving Sleep Apnea. https://survivingsleepapnea.com/do-you-have-to-use-a-cpap-machine-forever/

10 Tips to Help You Manage Irritation with Minoxidil. https://evolvedhair.com.au/10-tips-to-help-you-manage-irritation-with-minoxidil/

Unlocking The Potential Of Castor Oil For Prostate Health: A Natural Solution - ScienceSpace.blog. https://sciencespace.blog/castor-oil-prostate-health/

Why is Magnesium Essential for our Health? - BLUXOM Beauty Products. https://bluxom.com/blog-magnesium/

Tight or Sore Back? Loosen up at Forest Hills! - Forest Hills Rehab. https://foresthillsrehab.com/2024/02/12/loosen-up-tight-back/

# 132 | REFERENCES

Intermittent Fasting and Its Impact on Sperm Health and Male Fertility | CapScore. https://www.capscoretest.com/blogs/male-fertility-resources/intermittent-fasting-and-its-impact-on-sperm-health-and-male-fertility

Foods and Nootropics for Peak Brain Performance | Dietitian Nutritionist. https://teamnutrition.ca/blog-nutritionist-dietitian/foods-and-nootropics-peak-brain-performance

patientattitude.com | Top 10 Anti-Inflammatory Foods That Help Arthritis Symptoms. https://patientattitude.com/anti-inflammatory-foods-that-help-arthritis-symptoms

How Good Nutrition Boosts Your Wellness in 6 Ways. https://doms2cents.com/how-good-nutrition-boosts-your-wellness-in-6-ways/

The Ultimate Guide to the Best Post-Workout Recovery Drink & How to Incorporate It into Your Morning Meal. https://bangkok101-ca.com/the-ultimate-guide-to-the-best-post-workout-recovery-drink-how-to-incorporate-it-into-your-morning-meal

Navigating the Emotional Rollercoaster of Modern Life - My Framer Site. https://www.sagradaintegration.com/blog/navigating-the-emotional-rollercoaster-of-modern-life

The Rock Surprised Everyone When He Revealed His Daily Diet Habits And Is Forced To Consume More Than 9,000 Calories A Day - Celebrity. https://bestcelebrityzone.com/the-rock-surprised-everyone-when-he-revealed-his-daily-diet-habits-and-is-forced-to-consume-more-than-9000-calories-a-day/

Obese Scooter : Revolutionize Your Mobility - I'm Health Fit. https://www.iamhealthfit.com/obese-scooter/

loan | ifvod. https://ifvod.co/loan/

9 Substitutes for Tahini. https://asoothingliving.com/substitutes-for-tahini/

Sex drive boosted by hormone kisspeptin in trials - Lounge - Schizophrenia.com. https://forum.schizophrenia.com/t/sex-drive-boosted-by-hormone-kisspeptin-in-trials/291037

Tips Archives - RA Balance Bahamas. https://rabalancebahamas.com/tag/tips/

Pro-Dynabol (Methandienone) | Buy Anabolics Online | Rx Anabolics. https://www.rxanabolics.com/pd/198/pro-dynabol--methandienone-

Buy Best Black Seed/Cumin Oil Online at Cheap Price – Incense Pro. https://www.incensepro.com/products/black-seed-cumin-oil

Add a few drops of essential oil to the vacuum cleaner filter, it will spread the fragrance throughout the home when you are vacuuming. - Orania Website. https://www.orania.co.nz/?attachment_id=22521

Learn to live your best life at the Ladner Pioneer Library - Delta Optimist. https://www.delta-optimist.com/in-the-community/learn-to-live-your-best-life-at-the-ladner-pioneer-library-6397077

Book Marketing for Authors: Growing Your Author Platform. https://amzbookpublishing.com/book-marketing-for-authors-platform/

Discover the Role of Family Doctors in Senior Well-Being. https://www.elitecare-hc.com/blog/the-role-of-family-doctors-in-senior-well-being/

Are you ignoring the side effects of your daily caffeine intake?. https://jang.com.pk/en/16027-are-you-ignoring-the-side-effects-of-your-daily-caffeine-intake-news

Understanding Holistic Health: A Path to Wellness. https://www.holistic-health-101.com/post/understanding-holistic-health-a-path-to-wellness

Holistic Dentistry: Unlocking Better Smile, Health and Life. https://drshaunapalmer.ca/holistic-dentistry-better-smile-health-life-kelowna/

Unlocking the Secrets to Optimal Health and Fitness - angelahallstrom.com. http://www.angelahallstrom.com/unlocking-the-secrets-to-optimal-health-and-fitness.html

Hijama Therapy for Emotional and Mental Balance. https://www.huatuoclinic.com/hijama-therapy-for-emotional-and-mental-balance/

Kim, D., & Kwon, S. (2020). Vibrational stress affects extracellular signal-regulated kinases activation and cytoskeleton structure in human keratinocytes. PLoS One, 15(4), e0231174.

(2024). Australia : Significant progress on breakthrough cancer therapy. MENA Report, (), .

Layouni, R., Cao, T., Coppock, M., Laibinis, P., Weiss, S., & Weiss, S. (2021). Peptide-Based Capture of Chikungunya Virus E2 Protein Using Porous Silicon Biosensor. Sensors, 21(24), 8248.

Goldstein, J., & Cryer, B. (2015). Gastrointestinal injury associated with NSAID use: A case study and review of risk factors and preventative strategies. Drug, Healthcare and Patient Safety, 7(), 31-41.

Picuno, C., Godosi, Z., Santagata, G., Picuno, P., & Picuno, P. (2024). Degradation of Low-Density Polyethylene Greenhouse Film Aged in Contact with Agrochemicals. Applied Sciences, 14(23), 10809.

## REFERENCES WITH LINKS

The Forgotten Side of Medicine, October 12, 2024
The Forgotten Side of Medicine, September 29, 2024
X, Robert Kennedy Jr, October 25, 2024
The Forgotten Side of Medicine, October 20, 2024
The Forgotten Side of Medicine, September 15, 2024
The Forgotten Side of Medicine, October 20, 2024

## 134 | REFERENCES

The Forgotten Side of Medicine, November 17, 2024
The Forgotten Side of Medicine, September 15, 2024
The Forgotten Side of Medicine, November 10, 2024
Amazon, The DMSO Handbook for Doctors
The Forgotten Side of Medicine, October 12, 2024, comment
The Forgotten Side of Medicine, October 12, 2024, comment
The Forgotten Side of Medicine, December 9, 2024, comment
The Forgotten Side of Medicine, October 29, 2024, comment
The Forgotten Side of Medicine, October 29, 2024, comment
The Forgotten Side of Medicine, October 12, 2024, comment
The Forgotten Side of Medicine, November 18, 2024, comment
The Forgotten Side of Medicine, November 18, 2024, comment
The Forgotten Side of Medicine, October 13, 2024, comment
The Forgotten Side of Medicine, October 25, 2024, comment
The Forgotten Side of Medicine, October 13, 2024, comment
The Forgotten Side of Medicine, October 26, 2024, comment
The Forgotten Side of Medicine, October 26, 2024, comment
The Forgotten Side of Medicine, October 26, 2024, comment
The Forgotten Side of Medicine, October 30, 2024, comment
The Forgotten Side of Medicine, November 7, 2024, comment
The Forgotten Side of Medicine, November 14, 2024, comment
The Forgotten Side of Medicine, November 18, 2024, comment
The Forgotten Side of Medicine, November 8, 2024, comment
The Forgotten Side of Medicine, December 1, 2024
The Forgotten Side of Medicine, October 12, 2024, comment
The Forgotten Side of Medicine, October 14, 2024, comment
The Forgotten Side of Medicine, October 26, 2024, comment
The Forgotten Side of Medicine, October 12, 2024, comment
The Forgotten Side of Medicine, October 13, 2024, comment
The Forgotten Side of Medicine, November 18, 2024, comment
The Forgotten Side of Medicine, October 29, 2024, comment
The Forgotten Side of Medicine, October 13, 2024, comment
The Forgotten Side of Medicine, November 18, 2024, comment
The Forgotten Side of Medicine, November 18, 2024, comment
The Forgotten Side of Medicine, November 18, 2024, comment
The Forgotten Side of Medicine, December 9, 2024, comment
The Forgotten Side of Medicine, November 7, 2024, comment
The Forgotten Side of Medicine, October 13, 2024, comment
The Forgotten Side of Medicine, December 9, 2024, comment
The Forgotten Side of Medicine, October 19, 2024, comment

# REFERENCES | 135

The Forgotten Side of Medicine, December 9, 2024, comment
The Forgotten Side of Medicine, November 26, 2024, comment
The Forgotten Side of Medicine, November 18, 2024, comment
The Forgotten Side of Medicine, October 26, 2024, comment
The Forgotten Side of Medicine, November 8, 2024, comment
The Forgotten Side of Medicine, November 8, 2024, comment
The Forgotten Side of Medicine, October 17, 2024, comment
The Forgotten Side of Medicine, October 17, 2024, comment
The Forgotten Side of Medicine, October 17, 2024, comment
The Forgotten Side of Medicine, December 9, 2024, comment
The Forgotten Side of Medicine, December 3, 2024, comment
Amazon, The Persecuted Drug: The Story of DMSO
Amazon, The DMSO Handbook for Doctors
The Forgotten Side of Medicine, December 9, 2024, comment
The Forgotten Side of Medicine, December 9, 2024, comment
The Forgotten Side of Medicine, November 18, 2024, comment
The Forgotten Side of Medicine, December 9, 2024, comment
The Forgotten Side of Medicine, December 9, 2024, comment
The Forgotten Side of Medicine, October 12, 2024, comment
The Forgotten Side of Medicine, October 29, 2024, comment
The Forgotten Side of Medicine, October 12, 2024, comment
The Forgotten Side of Medicine, November 26, 2024, comment
The Forgotten Side of Medicine, November 7, 2024, comment
The Forgotten Side of Medicine, November 26, 2024, comment
The Forgotten Side of Medicine, October 13, 2024, comment
The Forgotten Side of Medicine, December 9, 2024, comment
The Forgotten Side of Medicine, October 13, 2024, comment
The Forgotten Side of Medicine, December 9, 2024, comment
The Forgotten Side of Medicine, November 27, 2024, comment
The Forgotten Side of Medicine, December 9, 2024, comment
Scientific Reports Volume 8, Article number: 4947 (2018)
The Forgotten Side of Medicine, December 1, 2024
The Forgotten Side of Medicine, September 15, 2024
The Forgotten Side of Medicine, September 29, 2024
Journal of the Korean Ophthalmological Society: 556-570, 2002
Fed Proc 1965; 24:214
Surg Forum. 1964:15:475-7
The Persecuted Drug: The Story of DMSO (Archived)
Klinische Wochenschrift, 01 Oct 1966, 44(19):1151-1152
Ger. Med. Mon., 12: 443-4 (Sept. 1967)

J. Invest. Dermatol., 52: 277-9 (Mar. 1969)
Klinische Wochenschrift, 01 Oct 1966, 44(19):1151-1152
Med. Radiol.; (USSR); Journal Volume: Jun 01, 1978 23:6
Med Radiol (Mosk). 1974 Nov;19(11):66-8
Yeungnam University (2002)
Annals of the New York Academy of Sciences, 141: 428-436
Otolaryngol Head Neck Surg 1994:110: 228-31
Plast Reconstr Surg. 1968 Jan;41(1):64-70
Aesthet Surg J. 2005 Mar-Apr;25(2):201-9
Otolaryngol Head Neck Surg. 1994 Feb;110(2):228-31
Plast Reconstr Surg. 2007 Dec;120(7):1819-1822
Journal of Investigative Dermatology, Volume 62, Issue 1, January 1974, Pages 51-53
Scandinavian Journal of Plastic and Reconstructive Surgery, Volume 4, 1970 - Issue 1
Cir. Vol. 91 No. 5 Ciudad de México September/October 2023
Genetics and Molecular Research 14 (4): 18160-18171 (2015)
Plastic and Reconstructive Surgery 49(1): Pages 109-110, January 1972
Annals of Plastic Surgery 11(3): Pages 223-226, September 1983
Plast Reconstr Surg. 2007 Dec;120(7):1819-1822
Aesthet Surg J. 2005 Mar-Apr;25(2):201-9
Clinical Surgery, 1985
Indian J Exp Biol. 1999 May;37(5):450-4
Klin Khir (1962). 1985 Mar:(3):38-40
J Burn Care Rehabil. 1995 May-Jun;16(3 Pt 1):253-7
Eur Rev Med Pharmacol Sci. 2013 Oct;17(19):2571-7
Can J Ophthalmol. 1987 Feb;22(1):17-20
DMSO: The New Healing Power (Archived)
The Forgotten Side of Medicine, September 29, 2024
The Forgotten Side of Medicine, September 29, 2024
Ann N Y Acad Sci. 1975 Jan 27:243:403-7
Schweiz Rundsch Med Prax. 1972 Oct 17;61(42):1300-4
Ann N Y Acad Sci. 1975 Jan 27:243:403-7
Schweiz Rundsch Med Prax. 1972 Oct 17;61(42):1300-4
Schweiz Rundsch Med Prax. 1974 Apr 2;63(13):399-401
Amazon, The Persecuted Drug: The Story of DMSO
Amazon, Healing with DMSO: The Complete Guide to Safe and Natural Treatments for Managing Pain, Inflammation, and Other Chronic Ailments with Dimethyl Sulfoxide
Amazon, The Persecuted Drug: The Story of DMSO

The Forgotten Side of Medicine, October 25, 2024, comment
X, JanuarysBeeRescueOnRumble/MedicalAnthropologist, December 7, 2024
Annals of the New York Academy of Sciences, 141: 490-492
Br J Pharmacol. 2020; 177: 3327–3341
Spectrochimica Acta Part A: Molecular and Biomolecular Spectroscopy, Volume 196, 5 May 2018, Pages 344-352
Annals of the New York Academy of Sciences, 243: 257-268
Klin Khir (1962). 1988:(1):1-3
The Forgotten Side of Medicine, September 29, 2024
The Forgotten Side of Medicine, September 15, 2024
J Am Geriatr Soc. 1985 Jan;33(1):41-3
Ann N Y Acad Sci. 1975 Jan 27:243:408-11
Wounds UK 15(15):361-370
Annals of the New York Academy of Sciences, 243: 395-402
Zeitschrift fur Haut- und Geschlechtskrankheiten, 01 Sep 1967, 42(18):749-754
Ann N Y Acad Sci. 1967 Mar 15;141(1):478-83
Amazon, The DMSO Handbook for Doctors
Amazon, Healing with DMSO: The Complete Guide to Safe and Natural Treatments for Managing Pain, Inflammation, and Other Chronic Ailments with Dimethyl Sulfoxide
Annals of the New York Academy of Sciences, 141: 638-645
Voen Med Zh. 1986 Jun:(6):57-8
Voen Med Zh. 1986 Jun:(6):57-8
Voenno-meditsinskii Zhurnal, 01 Nov 1991, (11):33-34
Annals of the New York Academy of Sciences, 141: 638-645
Chinese Medical Journal, September 1975
Vestnik Dermatologii i Venerologii, 01 Jan 1989, (9):71-72
Dermatologica (1976) 152 (5): 316–320
The Forgotten Side of Medicine, December 1, 2024
Int J Dermatol. 1998 Dec;37(12):949-54
Amazon, DMSO: The True Story of a Remarkable Pain-Killing Drug
Deutsche Medizinische Wochenschrift (1946), 01 Nov 1968, 93(44):2102-2106
The Forgotten Side of Medicine, December 1, 2024
Amazon, The DMSO Handbook: A New Paradigm in Healthcare
The Forgotten Side of Medicine, October 14, 2024, comment
The Forgotten Side of Medicine, October 29, 2024, comment
Amazon, The DMSO Handbook for Doctors
American Board of Dermatology, What Is a Dermatologist?
CMS.gov, NHE Fact Sheet
The Commonwealth Fund, January 31, 2023

"How DMSO Revolutionizes Skin Care and Dermatology," analyzed by A Midwestern Doctor, was published on December 27, 2024, on Dr. Joseph Mercola's website.

Musaeus, C., Salem, L., Kjaer, T., & Waldemar, G. (2019). Microstate Changes Associated With Alzheimer's Disease in Persons With Down Syndrome. Frontiers in Neuroscience, (), n/a.

www.ingramcontent.com/pod-product-compliance
Lightning Source LLC
Chambersburg PA
CBHW070634030426
42337CB00020B/4012